Birthing Your Placenta

the third stage of labour

Dr Nadine Edwards

Dr Sara Wickham

Birthing Your Placenta: the third stage of labour
Fourth edition published 2018 by Birthmoon Creations
Avebury and Edinburgh
© 2018 Nadine Edwards and Sara Wickham
www.sarawickham.com

Nadine Edwards and Sara Wickham have asserted their moral right to be named as the authors of this work in accordance with the Copyright, Designs and Patents Act of 1988.

ISBN-10: 1999806441
ISBN-13: 978-1-9998064-4-6
Also available as an e-book

Cover design by Chris Hackforth and Sara Wickham

This book offers general information for interest only and does not constitute or replace individualised professional midwifery or medical care and advice. Whilst every effort has been made to ensure the accuracy and currency of the information herein, the authors accept no liability or responsibility for any loss or damage caused, or thought to be caused, by making decisions based upon the information in this book and recommend that you use it in conjunction with other trusted sources of information.

ABOUT THE AUTHORS

Dr Nadine Edwards PhD is a long-standing birth activist, educator, researcher and writer. She currently works at and is a Trustee at the Pregnancy and Parents Centre, Edinburgh. She is former Vice Chair of the Association for Improvements in the Maternity Services and is working on several books.

Dr Sara Wickham PhD, RM, MA, PGCert, BA(Hons) is a midwife, educator, writer and researcher who offers online courses and speaks at workshops and conferences around the world. You can find Sara online at www.sarawickham.com, and she also has a free monthly newsletter. Some of her work is shared at www.facebook.com/saramidwife and @DrSaraWickham

Also by Nadine Edwards

Birthing Autonomy: women's experiences of planning home births
Birthing Your Baby: the second stage
Untangling the Maternity Crisis (with Rosemary Mander and Jo Murphy-Lawless)

Also by Sara Wickham

Anti-D in Midwifery: panacea or paradox?
Appraising Research into Childbirth
Group B Strep Explained
Inducing Labour: making informed decisions
Midwifery Best Practice (volumes 1-5)
Sacred Cycles: the spiral of women's wellbeing
Vitamin K and the Newborn
What's Right For Me? Making decisions in pregnancy and childbirth
101 Tips for planning, writing and surviving your dissertation

Acknowledgements

We would like to offer our very sincere thanks to Annie Barnes, Beverley Beech, Gill Boden, Penny Champion, Gill Gyte, Chris Hackforth, Mavis Kirkham and Kirsten Small. Their contributions, support, thoughtful comments and generous sharing of their expertise have greatly improved this book.

Julie Frohlich has been our book's editor, as she has been for several others, and we are deeply grateful for her careful and considered thoughts.

As always, our work comes from the discussions we have with women, midwives, student midwives, birth educators, activists, doulas, doctors, researchers and others. Their thoughts and insights help us to write what we hope are informative and supportive publications for those involved with birth, whatever views they hold. Our book is anchored in what we hear and we have looked at research within the context of practice rather than the other way around. We hope this makes the book particularly relevant to both women giving birth and those caring for them and their babies. In offering this book to you, we want to extend our thanks to all of those whose thoughts, experiences and stories have helped us along the way.

Contents

x

Notes on language, terminology and international variation

Although this book is written in the UK, we are aware that we have many international readers; women, midwives and others. In order not to exclude readers from areas where practices, drugs or medications, terminology and experiences may be different, we offer a few notes below as a quick guide to translation. The UK terms are explained throughout the text of the book.

- Uterotonic drugs are known in some areas as ecbolic drugs.
- Syntocinon is also known as Pitocin and this is the drug to which people are referring when they say synthetic oxytocin.
- Ergometrine is also known as Methergine and Ergonovine.
- Misoprostol goes by the brand name Cytotec in some areas.
- Carbetocin is also known as Duratocin and Pabal.

Physiological birth of the placenta is sometimes referred to as 'passive' or 'expectant' management of the third stage of labour. Throughout this book, however, we have talked more about the birth of the placenta rather than the third stage, especially when we are talking about the birth of the placenta under natural circumstances. We also often use the word 'born' rather than 'delivered' when we write about the placenta. We use such terms (a) because we feel it is important to acknowledge that it is a woman who gives birth to her baby and placenta (whereas 'management' is something that is done to women by others), and (b) because the artificial division of labour into stages that has emerged as part of the medical view of childbirth is not necessarily representative of how women themselves experience this journey. Furthermore, a number of people, including Michel Odent (1998a, 1998b) have pointed out that a physiological process does not need to be 'managed'. We will continue to look at elements of this discussion throughout the book.

It is, of course, in the privileged context of an affluent society where we have the means to treat excessive bleeding that this book is written. While describing our country as affluent however, we want to acknowledge that significant and growing inequalities impact upon pregnancy and birth experiences and outcomes (Tinson *et al* 2016). We also acknowledge that approaches to and treatment of the birth of the placenta may be different in middle and low income countries where birth may be less safe overall because of wars, women's status and role and the impact of poverty. This might result in poor health, lack of shelter, no access to medical help if needed, lack of even the most basic drugs and medicines, questionable practices or even inappropriate and outdated medical technology and interventions. Any or all of these can predispose women to excessive bleeding, which too often results in severe morbidity or death. While global inequalities are the real challenge, in the meantime it is crucial to continue to carry out research on which drugs and practices safely and effectively reduce bleeding.

"Care for pregnant women differs fundamentally from most other medical endeavours. 'Routine' care during pregnancy and birth interferes in the lives of healthy people, and in a process which has the potential to be an important life experience. It is difficult to imagine the extent to which our efforts might, for example, disturb the development of a confident, nurturing relationship between the mother and baby. The harmful effects we measure in randomised trials are limited to those we have predicted may occur. Sometimes after many years unexpected harmful effects surface only because they are relatively common, or striking in their presentation. Many unanticipated harmful effects probably never come to light.

For these reasons, interventions in pregnancy and childbirth need to be subjected to special scrutiny. Our guiding principle is to advise no interference in the process of pregnancy and childbirth unless there is compelling evidence that the intervention has worthwhile benefits for the mother and/or her baby – only then is there a good chance that benefits will outweigh both known adverse effects and those which may not have been thought of."

(Hofmeyr *et al* 2008: xiii)

Introduction

The birth of the placenta is part of the awesome journey from woman to mother. For most women or parents it follows closely on from the particularly precious moment when they meet their baby for the first time face to face; *"...there are emotional, physiological, bacteriologic, hormonal and spiritual exchanges between the mother and the infant during this special time"* (Mercer & Erickson-Owens 2010: 82).

In many cultures, the placenta itself is seen as an important and sometimes sacred organ, although it is also important to note that there are very differing perspectives on the significance, meaning and implications of this part of the journey of childbirth (Jordan 2017).

This book is for parents, midwives, doulas, childbirth educators, students and others who would like to know more about the birth of the placenta, why there are ongoing discussions about the benefits and drawbacks of medically managing the third stage of labour or letting nature take its course, and what research and experience can tell us about the birth of the placenta and related issues.

The third stage of labour is usually defined in textbooks as the period immediately following the baby's birth until the placenta and membranes have been born (Rankin 2017). Physiologically, it involves the hormone oxytocin, which is produced naturally by a woman's body and is intimately linked with labour and birth (Uvnäs Moberg 2003, 2011, Buckley 2009, 2015). Over the past decades, pharmacists have also developed synthetic forms of oxytocin which are commonly used within maternity care, although the synthetic form of oxytocin can interfere with a woman's ability to produce her own natural oxytocin (Foureur 2008). Oxytocin works by making the woman's uterus (womb) contract during labour, which brings about the birth of her baby. As the baby is born, a further surge of oxytocin brings about the birth of the placenta. The woman continues to produce oxytocin after birth (especially when she is able to cuddle and/or breastfeed her baby skin to skin) and this oxytocin helps to keep her uterus contracted and blood loss controlled. In a natural placental birth, there is no interference with the process and the placenta is birthed by the woman's own efforts. The amount of time that this takes varies from woman to woman, and we look at this in chapters 3 and 4.

A number of midwives have described the significance of this time. Jenny Sleep wrote in 1989 that the *"activity and excitement accompanying the birth of the baby are replaced by the parents' quiet and wondrous contemplation of their offspring. The focus shifts from the mother's concentrated exertions to the miracle of the newborn. There is a sense of emotional and physical relief"* (209).

Many women similarly describe experiencing this part of their birth journey as particularly special:

"It is hard to describe those first moments - such a mixture of joy and wonder and relief and curiosity about this new baby in your arms. And almost instantly it becomes hard to believe that they were ever in your tummy!" Joanna (Pregnancy and Parents Centre)

"I would say that nothing could have really prepared me for how wonderfully amazing it was to give birth to Finlay and finally hold him in my arms after 9 months of excited anticipation. If I could re-live that day tomorrow, I would do it in a second because it was such an astounding time. I would like to be able to go back and savour each moment again. Although I had been told by other people, I hadn't truly appreciated the miracle of creating a person, which continues to amaze me, and the overwhelming love you feel for them." Ros (Pregnancy and Parents Centre)

"Meeting our little girl was amazing; time seemed to stand still. She was a lot pinker and louder than I'd expected, and felt so fragile. I held her very close and wrapped her up in my arms – it was wonderful" Mel (Pregnancy and Parents Centre)

However, as much as this is a wondrous time for parents

as they meet their new baby, caregivers also see the birth of the placenta as a time when they need to be especially attentive, and this is because of the potential for excessive bleeding during the birth of the placenta. Evidence of this concern can be seen through subsequent editions of midwifery and related textbooks (Sleep 1993, McDonald 1999, Fraser & Cooper 2003, 2009, Rankin 2017). Such bleeding is less common in high-income countries, but when it does happen, it can be serious (WHO 2012, Knight *et al* 2017).

It is because of this concern that, increasingly, women have been advised to have 'active management of the third stage of labour' (sometimes abbreviated to AMTSL) for the birth of their placenta. The authors of the Cochrane review on this topic (Begley *et al* 2015) offer a useful definition. However, as we will discuss throughout the book, a number of aspects of this practice have been challenged and things are now changing.

"Active management of the third stage involves three components: 1) giving a drug (a uterotonic) to contract the uterus; 2) clamping the cord early (usually before, alongside, or immediately after giving the uterotonic), and this is before cord pulsation stops; 3) traction is applied to the cord with counter-pressure on the uterus to deliver the placenta (controlled cord traction). Specific ways the three components are used often vary. Mixed management uses some, but not all, of the three components." (Begley *et al* 2015).

Yet, while there is certainly a need for watchfulness, as excessive bleeding after birth can be a major source of maternal morbidity (illness) and even mortality (death), this level of bleeding is not usual and occurs in only a small proportion of healthy women who have had straightforward births. There is no way of eradicating all risk and many people believe the decision to enable the placenta to birth naturally is a reasonable one when labour and birth have been straight-forward, particularly where the equipment and medications to treat any excessive bleeding are available; and in the case of a home birth, where a hospital is accessible if necessary.

3

We do however have the disadvantage that birth in most parts of the affluent world has become increasingly medicalised, and some women and babies experience the consequences of the overuse of medication and medical procedures, which may have both known and unknown repercussions. One consequence of the medicalisation of birth is that interference with physiology at any time during labour and birth can mean that a woman is more likely to bleed during the birth of the placenta. For this reason, if labour and birth haven't been straightforward, active management decreases the likelihood of excessive bleeding during and after the birth of the placenta. Active management is also advised if women have a risk factor which makes them more likely to bleed during the birth of the placenta. One example of this is having a pre-existing bleeding disorder, and we will discuss such risk factors further in chapter 4. Like most interventions, active management of the third stage of labour carries risks and side effects as well as benefits, as we will also discuss in chapter 4.

The birth of the placenta is often accompanied by a significant level of fear. Generalised fear around the birth of the placenta is not always helpful, logical or in the best interests of mother and child. It does not always enable the birth attendant to focus on the woman and baby, or enable the woman to celebrate the birth of a new family member, which is so essential (Crowther 2015). Fear can also have an impact on a woman's ability to produce her own oxytocin for labour and birth. For women's bodies to produce the oxytocin they need to birth the placenta, they need to be in an environment where they feel safe and secure. Women need a trusted caregiver and a private space where they will not be inappropriately interrupted during labour and birth (Schmid 2005, Gurnsey & Davies 2010, Hastie 2011, Uvnäs Moberg 2011, Buckley 2009, 2015).

This book is intended to help women, midwives, doulas, childbirth educators, students and others understand more about the birth of the placenta and the different approaches that may be taken. It is divided into several chapters. Chapter 1 discusses the historical background to the birth of the placenta and introduces the different approaches to its management. Chapter 2 introduces the placenta and looks at the question of who it belongs to. Chapter 3 details the physiological birth of the placenta and a number of related issues and in chapter 4 we describe active management of the birth of the placenta, consider the situations in which this might be advised and look at the various drugs and interventions which may form a part of this. Chapter 5 looks at the research which has compared the different approaches and chapter 6 offers a discussion on the wider issues relating to this topic and also discusses women's decision making. The final section of the book offers references.

Nadine Edwards and Sara Wickham.
Edinburgh, Scotland. Summer 2018.

1. Historical background

It is impossible to know for sure how women birthed their placentas in ancient times and whether those who supported them intervened routinely (for instance with the use of herbs or physical manoeuvres) or simply supported women in their own efforts unless problems arose. We know that age-old beliefs exist in some cultures in relation to the meaning of the placenta and the rituals surrounding it. Some of these rituals still exist today, while others have been created more recently (Vincent-Priya 1991, 1992, Kitzinger 2000, Jordan 2017). We do not know whether, how and when ancient women separated themselves from their babies by biting or cutting the umbilical cord. Some people suggest that we should look at the behaviours of other mammals to gain an indication of this. Not everybody agrees with this, as humans live in a very different cultural context from other mammals. In any case, there is variation within the animal kingdom.

As beliefs about nature, science and the world in general began to change and people thought they could improve upon nature, women's bodies and birth were seen as unreliable processes to be managed and controlled (Murphy-Lawless 1998). These beliefs resulted in the development of tools and practices that enabled medical men to become more involved in childbirth from the 18th and 19th centuries onwards and, from this point on, more and more women found that their baby's birth was medically managed.

The vast majority of medical practices that exist in relation to the birth of the placenta today have become routine in high-income countries. It is likely that, as Murphy-Lawless' (1998) work suggests, these are partly based on the belief that women's bodies cannot be trusted, rather than on a good understanding of the physiology of placental birth. In many maternity services, the level of intervention is so high that third stage interventions are often needed because of earlier interference in the physiology of labour and birth. Such intervention can render a woman's body unable to secrete the natural oxytocin needed to birth the placenta safely.

The discovery of a fungus found on rotting rye (ergot), was one of the key developments in the history of the management of the birth of the placenta. It was initially discovered that cows who ate this fungus were more likely to miscarry their calves. We thus learned that ergot works very quickly and effectively to make the uterus contract. However, while midwives in the 17th and 18th centuries used ergot to treat bleeding after birth, they did so cautiously because it could also cause spasms of the blood vessels which could lead to gangrene (Inch 1989).

According to van Dongen & de Groot (1995), ergot's ability to hasten birth was documented as early as 1582, but this substance was (and still is) known to be a cause of uterine rupture, so from about 1828 it was used only as a means of stopping bleeding after birth. Dudley and Moir isolated ergometrine in 1932 (van Dongen & de Groot 1995, Inch 1989) and by 1935 the new water-soluble form of ergot was developed into a pharmaceutical product. Despite its side effects, ergometrine began to be used more frequently as a routine 'just in case' measure to prevent excessive bleeding rather than as an individualised treatment for women experiencing excessive bleeding. For more detailed information about its history see Inch 1989, van Dongen & de Groot 1995, Baskett 2000, Aflaifel & Weeks 2012.

The 1950s saw the advent of a synthetic, oxytocic drug called Syntocinon, which was hailed as a better alternative because it was thought that ergometrine could cause the lower part of the uterus to contract tightly around the placenta, preventing it from coming out. This is called a retained placenta (Inch 1989, Begley 1990a). However, Syntocinon was not considered to be as effective as ergometrine, and the 1960s saw the development of Syntometrine, a medication which combined Syntocinon and ergometrine. Both Syntocinon and Syntometrine are still in use, although Syntocinon has become the more popular first-line drug for the management of the third stage in recent years, as we will discuss later. Ergometrine is also used in addition in some circumstances. A range of other drugs and medications to prevent or treat postpartum bleeding has been developed and researched, as we discuss in chapter 4.

Changes in the treatment of the umbilical cord occurred along with the development of drugs. 'Early' or immediate cord clamping and cutting of the cord became widespread and practices developed which involved pulling on the cord as a way of removing the placenta more quickly. Pulling on the cord carries a risk of inverting the woman's uterus. The term 'an inverted uterus' describes what happens when the uterus turns inside out and comes down into the woman's vagina. Sometimes, part of the uterus protrudes from the vagina. This is extremely painful and can lead to maternal shock with a rapid drop in blood pressure. Therefore, the technique of pulling on the cord was paired with a technique called guarding the uterus, to prevent the woman's uterus from inverting. In this manoeuvre, practitioners support the woman's uterus in place by putting one hand firmly on the woman's abdomen in front of her uterus while applying traction to the cord with the other. There is considerable concern that these interventions may have exacerbated problems during the third stage of labour, which we discuss in chapter 4 (Botha 1968, Inch 1989, Dunn 1991, Dunn 2004, Mercer *et al* 2008, Buckley 2009, 2015, Mercer & Erikson-Owens 2010, Begley *et al* 2015).

It has been suggested that one reason that immediate clamping and cutting of the cord became popular was so that the baby could be removed from the bed and the attendants could focus on the mother 'unhindered' (Inch 1989). It is also thought that the practice of double clamping the cord was developed because the quantity of blood escaping from the placental end of the cut cord could make a mess (Inch 1989). In one of the earliest comprehensive reviews of third stage management, Sally Inch (1989) quotes Montgomery's view that these interventions might be due to the fact that:

"As the physician became more skilful with the use of haemostats, scissors and ligatures, the umbilical cord presented an inviting site for surgical procedures, and the present custom of immediate severance and immediate ligation of the cord followed. Ligation of the cord makes it possible to get babies and mothers out of the delivery room more rapidly, just as low forceps contribute to more rapid care. Whether they have added to the ultimate welfare of the newborn is a question" (Montgomery in Inch 1989: 166).

Montgomery's question continues to be pertinent and could still be asked about many aspects of maternity care. Despite the concerns that have been raised about routine active management of the third stage of labour, there has been a consensus in obstetric practice that it is necessary and desirable for all birthing women, in order to facilitate the expulsion of their placenta and prevent excessive bleeding after birth. Thus recent research and discussion have tended to focus only on drugs and interventions during the birth of the placenta. For example, which oxytocic drug to use, when and how much of the drug to use, whether controlled cord traction (pulling on the cord) is a useful element of this package of intervention, the impact of maternal effort (the woman pushing her placenta out) and fundal pressure (pressing on the woman's uterus). Less attention has been paid to what measures, if any, might reduce the likelihood of too much bleeding occurring in the first place. Midwives and others have suggested that such measures might include good nutrition to support the woman's health and the growth of a healthy baby and placenta, appropriate birthing environments and the presence of skilled and woman-centred birth attendants.

This is one area in which our thinking is significantly evolving. As we will discuss in later chapters, research evidence has highlighted a number of new findings in relation to the various components of an actively managed third stage. In addition, while current guidelines in many high-income countries support active management of the third stage of labour, they generally recommend that, *"If a woman at low risk of postpartum haemorrhage requests physiological management of the third stage,* [practitioners should] *support her in her choice."* (NICE 2017a: 1:14:11). The Cochrane review on this topic (Begley *et al* 2015) raises important questions about the routine use of actively managed third stage for healthy women who have had normal labours and births and who are not likely to bleed excessively after birth.

2. Introducing the placenta

When a woman conceives, the fertilised egg travels down her fallopian tube and implants in the wall of her uterus. Many complex processes take place and ultimately the egg forms into a growing baby with a placenta that is attached to the woman's uterine wall. The placenta enables the transfer of nutrients from the woman to her baby and the removal of waste products that the baby does not need. In nearly all cases, the egg embeds away from the woman's cervix (the neck of her uterus) so that the placenta is well away from her cervix and her baby can be born vaginally. Women who have ultrasound scans between 16 and 24 weeks are often told that their placenta is low. However, the uterus undergoes change and growth during pregnancy and most placentas will not be near the woman's cervix at the end of pregnancy (Heller *et al* 2014). Placenta praevia, where the placenta is covering all or part of the woman's cervix is very rare and affects around 5 in 1000 pregnancies (Cresswell *et al* 2013).

The placenta is a beautifully evolved organ and the complex physical relationship between the woman, baby and placenta means that the mother's blood and the baby's blood do not directly mix during pregnancy or birth. The structures and mechanisms that develop in the woman's uterus and placenta to prevent the mixing of blood also have a role in the physiological birth of the placenta, which we will discuss in the next chapter.

The fully grown placenta is roughly the size of a dinner plate. It usually weighs about a sixth of the baby's weight and the average umbilical cord – which connects the baby to its placenta - is around 50cm long. During the later stages of pregnancy, the volume of the woman's blood flowing through the maternal placental site in any one minute is 500-800ml (Rankin 2017). The placenta provides the baby with oxygen and other substances while it is in its mother's uterus and during the first few minutes after birth.

One of the more interesting things that we have learned over the years is that midwives noticed that following a physiological placental birth, the surface of the placenta that was attached to the woman's uterus appears smooth and shiny. Where active management of the third stage has been used, the placental surface appears dull and rough.

Who does the placenta belong to?

Over the next three chapters, we are going to talk about different aspects of placental birth and different ways of birthing the placenta. We will then look at some of the research relating to this area. However, we first want to address a key issue which comes up time and time again when we talk to women: the question of who the placenta belongs to and what happens to it after the birth.

Many women are unaware that the placenta is their property, but most are not consulted, during pregnancy, labour or birth, about what they would like to happen to their placenta. Many midwives will offer a woman and her partner the chance to see the placenta after birth, but the question of what happens to it is not usually discussed. Somewhat ironically, and perhaps because this topic is not often discussed in pregnancy, some women are quite surprised when they are offered the chance to see their placenta after the birth. Occasionally women are distressed to learn after its disposal that they could have kept their placenta.

In certain circumstances, caregivers may suggest that a woman's placenta is examined by a pathologist at the hospital because this can sometimes give useful information about her pregnancy and baby. For instance, examination may help determine whether twins are identical or non-identical.

In the past, placentas were sold by hospitals, health authorities/boards or health management organisations to be used in cosmetics. No matter whether women birth in hospital or at home, their placentas are now usually disposed of by incineration. Sometimes placentas are used in research. But we feel it important that readers know that every woman has the right to keep her placenta and, if she births somewhere other than her own home, to take her placenta home with her if she wishes to do so. On a practical level, if you are giving birth in a birth centre or hospital or packing a bag in case of hospital transfer, any woman who wishes to take her placenta home should take an appropriate container with her. A one litre plastic tub or box is a good receptacle, and it can also be useful to take a few large plastic bags, such as bin bags (trash bags), to prevent any leakage during transport.

There is a growing interest both in the social and spiritual aspects of the placenta as an extraordinary organ which nourishes the baby during pregnancy, and in the rituals associated with it (Vincent-Priya 1992, Lim 2015, Jordan 2017). Some women decide they would like to keep their placenta attached to their baby until it falls off naturally; a practice known as lotus birth. We discuss this and other placenta rituals in chapter 6.

3. Physiological birth of the placenta

There is growing evidence that when labour and birth have been normal, there is usually no need to induce or accelerate the birth of the placenta (Odent 1998b, Dixon *et al* 2009, Fahy *et al* 2010, Buckley 2015). The term 'normal birth' is a contentious one, and is defined differently in the research which looks at this, but there is general agreement that it describes a birth which began spontaneously, progressed without the use of synthetic hormones or pain relieving drugs such as opiate or epidural analgesia and without the assistance of instruments (such as forceps or ventouse). Ideally, the woman also remains undisturbed and is free to move as she pleases. Another way of looking at this was offered by the Royal College of Midwives (RCM 2008) when they suggested that physiological birth of the placenta '*…can be seen as a logical ending to a normal labour'.*

When we talk about physiological birth of the placenta, we mean that the placenta is born without interference. Drugs are not given, the cord is not immediately clamped and cut and controlled cord traction is not used, so the placenta is born as a result of maternal effort, and sometimes it literally falls out with no effort; we discuss controlled cord traction further in chapter 5. The birth of the placenta occurs at the same time that parents meet their new baby and begin to form a loving relationship. The birth of the placenta and the falling in love that happens between parents and baby are assisted by the presence of certain hormones. The most important of these hormones is oxytocin, which is also known as the 'hormone of love' (Odent 1998a, 1998b, 2002, Uvnäs Moberg 2011, Buckley 2015). Any approach to placental birth should therefore seek to minimise interference and, ideally, promote skin to skin contact which we now know is a crucial element of this journey (Schmid 2005, Hastie 2011). These things can optimise the release of oxytocin.

The anatomy and physiology of placental birth

When we look at the anatomy and physiology of the woman, baby and placenta, we can see how this supports physiological birth of the placenta. The uterine musculature is unique in its elasticity and its ability to expand and contract during and after pregnancy and birth. This elasticity is affected by the flow of oxytocin through a woman's body (Buckley 2015). It is the elastic nature of the woman's uterus that enables it to expand as the baby and placenta grow during pregnancy and to then reduce in size as the baby and placenta are born. A woman's uterine muscles tighten immediately after the birth of the baby and placenta. This tightening ensures that the part of the uterus to which the placenta was attached will be clamped down enough to prevent excessive bleeding in the first hours, days and weeks after birth. Under normal circumstances, the woman's uterus will remain contracted and will return to its non-pregnant size over the first few days and weeks after birth.

Once the baby has been born, the placenta usually begins to separate from the uterine wall. The placenta continues to function for a short time even after the baby and the placenta have been born. An obstetrician colleague describes this as happening *"in the same way that oxygen and carbon dioxide move in and out of the lungs even when you are holding your breath"* (Kirsten Small, personal correspondence 2018). The separation of the placenta happens very quickly in some women and more slowly in others, just as in other stages of labour. Disturbing the woman at any time during labour can slow or stop her labour, and many people have noticed that if a woman is disturbed around the time of birth, the separation and birth of the placenta can be much slower and may result in complications. This may be because adrenaline, the hormone produced in response to stress, interferes with the ability of the woman's body to produce the oxytocin that facilitates the birth of the placenta as well as the baby (Odent 1998a, Buckley 2009, 2015).

Researchers don't understand exactly how placental separation happens. It is generally thought that the placenta folds in on itself and the contracting upper part (or segment) of the uterus causes it to fall into the lower segment of the woman's uterus. Simultaneously the muscle fibres in the upper segment of her uterus (sometimes referred to as 'living ligatures') are able to clamp the exposed uterine blood vessels due to the pressure of the rapidly shrinking uterus. Meanwhile the woman's cervix remains open and, if she is upright, the placenta meets little resistance and passes into her vagina. It is then expelled, usually aided by gravity and the woman's pushing efforts (Kierse 1998), helped by the release of oxytocin in the mother (especially likely if her baby nuzzles or feeds at her breast).

Meanwhile, for the baby…

A number of changes occur as a baby is born and in the first minutes of its life which help it to adapt from life inside its mother's womb to life outside the womb. While in its mother's uterus, the baby's lungs are not expanding and breathing air. Because the baby's lungs have not yet inflated, they do not need as much blood circulation as they will do when the baby is born and begins to breathe air. At any given time, a relatively small amount of the unborn baby's blood circulates in its lungs (about 8-10 per cent). The placenta requires a constant flow of blood however, and a significant proportion of the baby's blood is circulating in the placenta throughout pregnancy (Mercer 2001).

The changes that the baby's body undergoes from being in the uterus (and getting oxygen from the placenta) and moving to what is called pulmonary circulation (where the baby uses its lungs to breathe and gain oxygen from air) occur when the baby takes its first breath or gasp (Mercer 2001, Mercer *et al* 2008, Mercer & Erickson-Owens 2010). The taking of this breath creates the need for the lung tissue to be filled with blood. At birth, the baby's first breaths will also expand its lungs so that they fill with air. From this point, the baby will be able to get oxygen from breathing. In order for this transition to happen most easily, the baby needs much more blood to flow to its lungs (Mercer 2001, Mercer *et al* 2008, Mercer & Erickson-Owens 2010).

In the past it was widely assumed that the baby only needed air for its lungs to expand and for it to begin to breathe on its own. However, researchers have been aware for several decades that babies adapt more easily and are healthier if their cords are not clamped immediately at birth (Mercer *et al* 2000). We now know that this is because the baby's circulating blood includes the blood that is in the placenta and that this blood is needed for this transition, which is why early cord clamping is detrimental. It is now clear that the transition the baby makes is more complex than was first thought and that the baby's dependence on the placenta does not end abruptly at birth.

The value of leaving the cord intact

"Another thing very injurious to the child is the tying and cutting of the navel string too soon: which should always be left till the child has not only repeatedly breathed but till all pulsation in the cord ceases. As otherwise the child is much weaker than it ought to be, a portion of blood being left in the placenta which ought to have been in the child." (Darwin 1801)

In days gone by, it would probably have been unnatural for a mother to sever the umbilical cord immediately, although common sense suggests that the timing and method of cord severing would be dependent on the circumstances and context in which a woman birthed. As we have already noted, we can't go back in time to see how our ancestors severed their babies' cords, but we know from the animal kingdom that there are a range of behaviours. In more recent times, maternity practitioners adopted the practice of clamping and then cutting the baby's umbilical cord soon after birth, thus separating the baby from its mother. But the nature and timing of this practice has been questioned and reconsidered in turn.

Here, we will begin by describing what happens if the baby's umbilical cord remains unclamped and intact for a while after birth. We will also explain what we know about how this is advantageous for the baby. As a slight (but we think important) aside, there hasn't been much interest in studying what happens in women's and babies' bodies if birth is not interfered with. Because of this, much of what we know about the advantages of waiting has come out of research studies looking at the disadvantages of immediate cord clamping. This is sadly not a unique situation. There are many other situations in maternity care where normal physiology is not well understood and in which we may well be causing more harm than good by interfering on a routine basis.

The transition to extrauterine life

As the mother and baby get to know each other in the minutes after birth, blood continues to flow between the baby and the placenta while the baby's body is adapting to life outside the womb. In the womb, the baby was in amniotic fluid and didn't need to breathe or eat as it received nourishment via the placenta. Once born, the baby needs to breathe air and ingest food and fluid in order to sustain itself as a separate person. The process of adapting to this new state is sometimes described as the transition to extrauterine life.

The umbilical cord continues to pulsate while the baby makes its transition, although midwives note that there is some variation in the length of time for which the cord pulsates. That is, some babies' cords seem to stop pulsating more quickly than others, but we don't yet know much about the relationship between being able to feel pulsation and whether blood flow is continuing to the baby. We have heard stories of babies who needed additional help establishing their breathing and whose cords pulsated for quite a while after they were born, and it is tempting to conclude that a protective mechanism may be at play here, but it is also important to note that most babies take a relatively short time to adapt to life outside the womb.

Some important things happen during this transition. Some of the baby's organs, including the lungs, gut and kidneys, are not used as much in the mother's uterus as they are outside her uterus, and these organs all need more blood after birth than before (Mercer *et al* 2008, Mercer & Erickson-Owens 2010, Hutchon 2012). In order not to draw upon blood which is needed elsewhere in the baby's body, blood is transferred from blood vessels in the cord and placenta to the baby in the moments after birth. Sometimes this is described or viewed as being 'extra' blood, but it is key to understand that this is a normal, expected and important part of birth. For this reason, it isn't helpful when people (or companies) use the term 'cord blood', as if this was an 'optional extra' which can be discarded or, as is now more common, collected for financial or other gain. This blood is the baby's blood and it has an important function in a baby's development.

For the same reason, there is currently some debate about the best terms to use when we talk or write about the timing of cord clamping. Many people use the term 'delayed', but this might suggest that cord clamping and cutting is happening too late when actually it is happening at the optimal time. Terms such as 'early' and 'late' are relative, but 'optimal', while better in some ways, isn't well-defined. Anthropologist Christine McCourt (personal correspondence 2018) has suggested using the term 'precipitate' to describe early cord clamping. This is helpful in that it implies that early cord clamping is overly hasty. As McCourt (2013) notes in her book on childbirth, midwifery and time, our language both shapes and is shaped by our worldview; and we can learn much more broadly and deeply when we step away from our everyday understandings and examine them more carefully.

In 2015, the Royal College of Obstetricians and Gynaecologists (RCOG) proposed the term 'deferred' as another alternative for describing the timing of clamping, but this hasn't yet been adopted into widespread use and this debate will probably continue for a while.

Evidence of the advantages of patience

The transfer of the blood that has been circulating in the placenta in the moments after birth is the main reason that it is important to allow time before clamping and cutting the baby's cord. Many practitioners are aware that the baby needs to be able to access its full complement of blood in order to support lung expansion and additional blood volume requirements from the placenta which occur as the first breaths of air are taken. If the cord is clamped immediately at birth, blood from the placenta cannot flow through it and this blood therefore cannot be used to support the process of lung expansion and respiration. Blood then has to be 'borrowed' from the rest of the baby's circulation in order for its lungs to become fully functioning, even though the baby's other vital organs also need blood to function fully and optimally (Mercer *et al* 2008, Mercer & Erickson-Owens 2010).

We are only really beginning to discover the myriad reasons why babies need to be able to access their full complement of blood before we interfere with the supply by clamping and cutting the cord. Our knowledge of this area has increased fairly rapidly over the past few years, although we still have a lot to learn. In 1974, Yao and Lind found that, when a baby received its full quota of blood, it was better able to maintain its haematocrit levels (ratio of red blood cells to total volume of blood). In the past, commentators knew that this quota of blood was important (Inch 1983) but it is only more recently that we have come to understand the implications of early cord clamping more fully.

The research in this area has now become more widely known and incorporated into practice. A number of studies have shown that allowing the cord to remain intact for a period of time confers significant advantages to the baby (Mercer & Erickson-Owens 2010, Hutchon 2012, Bhatt *et al* 2013, McDonald *et al* 2013, Mercer & Erickson-Owens 2014, Hooper *et al* 2015). Our current understanding is that allowing the cord to remain intact helps a baby to establish their breathing and circulation, which is particularly advantageous for babies who are compromised or born prematurely (Mercer & Erickson-Owens 2010). Allowing the cord to remain intact can lead to a reduction in breathing difficulties and less need for oxygen, ventilation and blood transfusion (Mercer 2001). Other benefits include an improvement in cardiac (heart) function (Bhatt *et al* 2013, Hooper *et al* 2015), an increase in the baby's iron stores (Chaparro *et al* 2006, Andersson *et al* 2011) and neurological advantages (Hutchon & Wepster 2014).

We know that later cord clamping can lead to a baby receiving almost a billion more stem cells (which have healing qualities) than if the cord is clamped and cut early (Mercer & Erickson-Owens 2010). Later cord clamping can also reduce the likelihood of severe infection (also known as sepsis) in pre-term babies (Mercer & Erickson Owens 2006, Mercer & Erickson Owens 2010). Hutchon (2016b) suggested that the intervention of immediate cord clamping may cause some babies to need to be resuscitated. Other studies show that babies whose cords are clamped earlier experience disadvantages. Mercer *et al* (2008) note that babies who experience immediate cord clamping are likely to have hypovolaemia (too little blood volume) and suggest that this can lead to the release of substances called inflammatory cytokines, which are associated with cerebral palsy.

While severing the baby's blood supply quickly and suddenly can have notable effects on some full-term babies, the effects can be even more detrimental in babies who are premature (particularly if born by caesarean section) or who are slow to breathe at birth (Dunn 1989, Mercer *et al* 2000, Mercer 2001, Mercer *et al* 2008, Mercer & Erickson-Owens 2010, 2014). In addition to all the impacts of a reduced circulating blood volume, red blood cells and stem cells that we have previously noted, pre-term babies are more likely than full-term babies to need additional oxygen, ventilation and blood transfusions and are more likely to suffer from intraventricular haemorrhage (a bleed in their brain), breathing difficulties, and sepsis.

Brocato *et al* (2016) showed that premature babies have less chance of needing a blood transfusion or of having an intraventricular haemorrhage if they are given time to access their full complement of blood. A number of hospitals are now buying and using equipment which enables staff to provide additional help (resuscitation) to premature or compromised babies while they remain alongside their mothers with their umbilical cords intact.

These benefits are summarised in systematic reviews and acknowledged in reviews looking at the 'management' of the birth of the placenta. In 2010, the Cochrane review comparing active management with physiological placental birth noted that about 20 per cent of a baby's blood volume is lost when the cord is clamped early (Begley *et al* 2010). This is also acknowledged in reviews on cord clamping, for instance where McDonald *et al* (2013) note Mercer's (2001) revelation that *"…placental transfusion can provide the infant with an additional 30% more blood volume and up to 60% more red blood cells."* The benefits of higher iron stores are experienced for several months after birth, even if the cord remains intact for only 1-3 minutes after birth (McDonald *et al* 2013). In both early and more recent studies, there is a bit of inconsistency in the actual amount of blood volume that babies are estimated to receive if the cord is left pulsating. We don't know why this is, although it is possible that this is a normal and natural variation in what happens if babies' bodies are allowed to determine their own needs.

Are there disadvantages to waiting?

The only known disadvantage to taking a more patient approach to cord clamping is that babies who experience later cord clamping are more likely to be diagnosed as needing phototherapy to treat jaundice. Physiological jaundice is not uncommon and it is caused by an excess of blood cells. These blood cells are broken down in the liver and one of the by-products is bilirubin. Babies are not always able to get rid of bilirubin quickly so it can build up, causing the yellowing of the skin which is the first sign of jaundice. Most jaundice passes without problems, but a few parents will be offered treatment for their baby if bilirubin levels rise above normal. The treatment usually involves the baby lying on a blanket or in a cot which contain special lights that help break down the bilirubin.

The current Cochrane review concludes that, *"A more liberal approach to delaying clamping of the umbilical cord in healthy term infants appears to be warranted, particularly in light of growing evidence that delayed cord clamping increases early haemoglobin concentrations and iron stores in infants. Delayed cord clamping is likely to be beneficial as long as access to treatment for jaundice requiring phototherapy is available."* (McDonald *et al* 2013).

This is an interesting finding and it raises some questions about whether this is truly problematic for a small number of babies and/or whether our current perceptions of what is normal in this area have been influenced by decades of practice in which cords were clamped and cut so soon after birth that babies were deprived of their full complement of blood. During an interview with Sharon Muza, paediatrician Mark Sloan helped put this finding into context: *"The apparent association between DCC* [delayed cord clamping] *and an increased need for phototherapy is a bit controversial. As pointed out by Dr. Judith Mercer, an expert on the benefits of delayed clamping, this concern is based largely on a single unpublished 1996 study performed by one of the Cochrane review's authors (McDonald). McDonald's study is one of only two of the nearly forty studies considered for inclusion in the current review that includes unpublished data; when that data is removed, the difference between groups loses significance."* (Muza 2017). Mercer *et al* (2017) subsequently published a small but interesting study in which they found no increase in jaundice in babies who had cord clamping delayed for five minutes after the birth.

Another recent study has thrown more light on the question of whether and how jaundice may be advantageous to babies. Hansen *et al* (2018) suggest that physiological jaundice may have an evolutionary role in protecting the baby against early-onset sepsis, which adds weight to the argument that the increased rate of jaundice may not be a problem, at least for the vast majority of babies. Specifically, their research showed that the additional bilirubin levels experienced by babies whose cords are not interfered with immediately after birth has antibacterial properties. They found a correlation between higher bilirubin levels and less growth of Group B Streptococcus (GBS) bacteria in a laboratory setting. This has implications for women who are considering GBS screening and treatment as well as for women who are considering their options for the birth of their placenta (Wickham 2018c).

Whether or not there is a slight increase in jaundice for babies who have later cord clamping, and whether or not this is somehow advantageous, commentators generally agree that waiting to clamp and cut the cord is beneficial and should be the default option. Mark Sloan added that, *"Conversely, there is no convincing argument in support of clamping the umbilical cord before a minute of age"* (Muza 2017).

How long should we wait?

If waiting is beneficial, then the next question is how long should we wait? The answer to that depends on how the woman wants the birth of her placenta to happen. If a woman decides to birth her placenta physiologically, then there isn't any need to rush to clamp and cut the cord. Some women and caregivers wait until the placenta is born before doing this, while others decide to do it after a few minutes, perhaps because the woman wants to move into a different position.

If the woman wants to have an actively managed placental birth, the cord is generally clamped and cut at birth. Nowadays it is more common to delay cord clamping for two to three minutes in tandem with administering a uterotonic. That is, the injection is given shortly after the baby is born but as it takes two to three minutes to take effect, the cord can be left intact during that time.

The WHO (2017) recommends that cord clamping should be delayed for one to three minutes after the birth although the quality of the evidence underpinning this recommendation was described as moderate. Guidelines in many countries now support deferred cord clamping as the norm (e.g. SOGC 2015, ACOG 2016, NICE 2017b, RANZCOG 2017), but we don't yet have clear evidence for the timing of this. The Cochrane review (McDonald *et al* 2013) cites a textbook (McDonald 2003) rather than a research study alongside the statement that most cords stop pulsating within two minutes of birth, and the studies which compared early with late cord clamping used a variety of different time frames, so it is not easy to draw conclusions from comparing their results. Some maternity care systems are, at least in theory, basing their guidelines on the WHO (2012) recommendation of waiting for between one and three minutes. In the UK, the RCOG published a Scientific Opinion Paper in 2015 which defined early cord clamping as before 30 seconds after birth and recommended defining deferred cord clamping as being at least two minutes after birth. The authors described clamping which occurred between 30 seconds and two minutes after birth as intermediate. Most of the benefits of delayed cord clamping that we have examined are gained within the first two minutes after birth (McDonald *et al* 2013, RCOG 2015). There may be other benefits that we have not yet thought about or researched.

We need more research in this area, in order to knowmore about the optimal timing of cord clamping. One complicating factor is the variations between the timing used in the studies which we have already mentioned. Much of the research is carried out on women who had active management of their third stage, so we don't know how the results apply to women who wish to give birth to their placentas physiologically. Another issue is that the authors of reviews do not always take into consideration the context of research trials and the situational and social factors which might have affected the outcomes. And, as we shall look at next, there are those who say that we need to look more broadly at the advantages of waiting and not focus only on the physical outcomes.

The social benefits of waiting

As we have seen, there are numerous physiological benefits of a more patient approach to cord clamping for healthy term babies, *"with virtually no risk of harm to mother and baby."* (Muza 2017).

Beyond the physical benefits of leaving the cord intact for a short while after birth, researchers have discussed the way in which early cord clamping leads to less 'protected' time for the mother and her baby (Mercer & Erickson-Owens 2010). Some people feel that there are social and psychological advantages for the mother and baby having undisturbed time before the cord is clamped and cut. This undisturbed time can enhance the relationship which begins to develop between the mother, her baby and her partner, if present. Any siblings or other family members present will also be meeting the baby for the first time.

The first hour or so after birth is a particularly awesome, miraculous, important, delicate and intense time of transition for mother, baby and family. If undisturbed, both mother and baby will continue to produce hormones that help them to form a strong, loving connection. This helps the woman to feel protective of her baby and, according to physiologist and midwife Verena Schmid (2005), it contributes to ongoing attachment patterns between mother and baby, between family and baby and in the baby's ongoing relationships as it moves through childhood into adulthood.

In a more relaxed setting where cord clamping and cutting are delayed, the mother and baby may be more likely to have skin to skin contact and the baby may nuzzle and begin to suckle at its mother's breast. This improves the baby's oxygen levels and lowers its heart rate (Mercer & Erickson-Owens 2010). Skin to skin cuddling also increases the flow of the hormone oxytocin, which helps the separation of the woman's placenta and is the main hormone of love (which Foureur (2008) notes was a term first used by Niles Newton) and bonding (Odent 1999, Schmid 2005). Babies nurtured this way have been shown to breastfeed for 10–12 days longer than those with early cord clamping (Mercer 2001).

In most cases, the umbilical cord is long enough that the baby can easily reach and be held at the woman's breast, or on or near her chest, even while the placenta is still in the uterus. But, as with many things, cord length can vary between babies and, occasionally, the cord is quite short. Sometimes, a midwife or doctor will give this as a reason to suggest cutting the cord quickly. But you can say that you want the cord to be left intact and hold the baby on your lap until the cord stops pulsating. The baby does not need to go to the breast immediately and in fact lots of women like to look at and explore their baby first (no matter what length the cord is) before they bring the baby to their chest for a cuddle.

Other benefits of waiting

A large systematic review (which we will consider in more depth in chapter 5) found that healthy women who have a physiological birth of their placenta are less likely to experience after pains, less likely to experience vomiting, less likely to need analgesia (pain relief) in the first hours after birth, and less likely to need to return to hospital because they are bleeding heavily in the days or weeks after birth. They are also less likely to have high blood pressure than women who had an actively managed third stage which includes uterotonics containing ergot compounds (Begley *et al* 2015). Furthermore, the woman's sense of confidence in her own body may be enhanced.

Some people have theorised that, particularly where a woman is having a physiological birth of her placenta, a more relaxed approach to cord clamping may also confer physical benefits in relation to the birth of the placenta itself. Dunn *et al* (1966) raised the possibility of the placenta being bulkier when fetal blood is prevented from passing to the baby. At the time of this research, it was suggested that early cord clamping might prolong placental separation due to fetal blood remaining in the placenta, which may delay contraction of the woman's uterus. Botha (1968) suggested that clamping the maternal end of the cord may interfere with placental separation and predispose a woman to greater blood loss; an idea which was noted by Levy (1990) and Rogers & Wood (1999). To our knowledge, none of these ideas has ever been the main focus of research.

A few researchers have also speculated about the possibility of feto-maternal transfusion (mixing of the baby and mother's blood) because of a larger volume of blood remaining in the placenta. One theory is that, as the uterus attempts to contract to expel the placenta, the pressure exerted can cause placental vessels to rupture, allowing fetal cells into the maternal system. This may be significant if the mother is Rhesus negative and her baby is positive (Lapido 1972, Prendiville & Elbourne 1989, Wickham 2001). Rogers *et al* (1998) considered this in their research but did not confirm an association.

We will look more closely at the question of cord clamping

and cutting in relation to actively managed placental birth in chapter 4.

How long does it take to birth a placenta?

There can be considerable variation in the length of time between the birth of the baby and the birth of the placenta when this occurs physiologically. Occasionally, the placenta is attached to the woman's uterus in such a way that it will not come away naturally. If this happens, or if a woman bleeds excessively, then intervention will be recommended. There has been debate over the years about the maximum safe length of time for the birth of the placenta. We know from correspondence with one of the researchers in the Hinchingbrooke third stage trial (Rogers *et al* 1998) that the decision to intervene after one hour is often a purely pragmatic one in busy maternity units (Jane Rogers 1999, personal communication). We discuss what happens in the event of retained placenta in chapter 4.

In an article summarising the views of midwives in relation to physiological placental birth, Davies (2011) wrote that, *"…in the vast majority of cases the placenta will arrive within 10-30 minutes, but if a longer period transpires it is not necessarily an immediate cause for concern."* Several of the midwives said they were happy to wait an hour or more as long as there were no problems and the woman was also happy to wait. These midwives' views are in accord with the UK NICE guidelines which state that, if a woman has physiological management (sic), a prolonged third stage of labour is diagnosed if the birth of the placenta has not occurred within 60 minutes of the birth (NICE 2017a: 1:14:3).

A study of women cared for by New Zealand midwives found that only 11.3 per cent of more than 16,000 women who had a physiological placental birth experienced a third stage of longer than 40 minutes (Dixon *et al* 2009). However, earlier work by Cronk and Flint (1989) proposed that up to ninety minutes could be normal for some women, and it is important to differentiate between what is average and situations which might be considered unusual but are still within the realms of safety and simply on the edge of the normal range. Many midwives have stories about extremes. One account describes a breech baby arriving unexpectedly at home, wearing its placenta like a "floppy hat" (Wesson 2006: 124), while other anecdotal accounts tell of the placenta being born many hours after the baby's birth.

Sometimes, there will be a concern that the birth of the placenta is taking too long. In this situation, the woman may be advised to have a uterotonic drug and possibly other components of active management. If there is concern that the placenta is attached in a problematic way, manual removal of the placenta may be suggested. We will discuss this in more depth in the last section in chapter 4.

Facilitating physiological birth of the placenta

Ideally, the women should be free to move into any position that she finds comfortable throughout labour and birth, including the birth of the placenta. The woman should be kept warm and comfortable, as higher levels of catecholamines (stress hormones) are associated with blood loss. The woman may produce catecholamines if she is too cool (Odent 1998b, Buckley 2015). Putting the baby skin to skin and perhaps to the mother's breast will stimulate her body to release oxytocin. Breast-feeding is not a prerequisite for physiological birth of the placenta: if the baby 'nuzzles' near its mother's breast or if she cuddles her baby, this will have a similar effect on the woman's oxytocin levels (Foureur 2008). Also, even if skin to skin cuddling is impossible for some reason, this does not preclude physiological birth of the placenta.

One of us (Sara) wrote an article sharing the views and experiences of midwives who had supported many women to have a physiological birth of their placenta (Wickham 2013).

These midwives emphasised the value of patience and facilitation when attending a physiological placental birth. As one of the midwives said, *"The work of the midwife after the baby is born is just to hold the space for love to happen. Don't let anybody interfere with this sacred and important moment in which love and interaction should happen. The interference can be from talking directly to the mother, other professionals, the mother not feeling comfortable, someone talking on the phone, someone trying to 'help' with breastfeeding and forcing the baby's mouth on the breast, and all of these can distract the mother from her baby instead of just being in the moment. So hold the space, protect the space of mother and baby so they can meet each other in their own time and rhythm."* (Wickham 2013).

However, the same midwives stressed that vigilance is also vital, noting that bleeding can occasionally happen quickly (Wickham 2013). If there is concern at any point, midwives are ready to act. Experienced midwives will be just as skilled in emergency measures to stop or treat bleeding when these are needed as they are in facilitating the hormones of birth when things are going well.

Midwives will look out for signs of placental separation and descent. If the midwife thinks that the birth of the placenta may be delayed, but that there is no concern about wellbeing, a number of things can be tried. Some of these are used to help with separation, and some with the actual birth of the placenta. Examples include nipple stimulation, changing position, suggesting that the woman tries to pass urine or asking the woman to cough or blow into or across the top of a bottle. A number of alternative remedies are used throughout the world.

Whether or not complications arise depends on a variety of factors. To some extent, the woman's general health and energy levels and whether or not she is genuinely anaemic can be important in determining how a woman will cope with excessive blood loss. Clearly, a major haemorrhage is going to be debilitating for any woman, regardless of her general health. We say 'genuinely' anaemic in the sentence above because, in many areas, the cut-off point which is used to diagnose anaemia does not take into account the fact that healthy women often have lower iron levels in later pregnancy. This is because their blood volume increases, and it is normal for haemoglobin to be diluted. We would encourage any women who is told that she is anaemic but who feels well to talk to an experienced practitioner about their individual situation and blood results.

The skill of those attending the birth in facilitating the physiological birth of the placenta, detecting developing problems, preventing or treating bleeding, protecting the woman from infection, detecting a retained placenta and preventing or treating shock are all equally important. Midwives often stress that labour and birth are social and emotional as well as physiological journeys. Just as in earlier phases of labour, emotional factors may delay the process and the woman may need patience and quietness to let her placenta go and make the final transition to motherhood (Edmunds 1998). It is also important that a woman does not feel 'observed' by those around her, as this can inhibit the flow of oxytocin and instead cause stress hormones to be released (Odent 1998b).

A key consideration is that, for a variety of reasons – including the fact that many hospitals encourage women to have an actively managed third stage – some midwives and doctors are neither comfortable nor experienced in helping women to birth their placenta naturally. Women often report that midwives attending births in women's homes, birth centres or midwifery-led units tend to be more likely and able to facilitate physiological placental birth.

How a woman feels during placental birth

As we have already noted, the way in which a birth unfolds has direct and indirect physical and emotional implications for the relationship between a mother and her baby, and can affect how the mother feels about herself for a long time afterwards. In this section, we want to look at how a woman might feel during the physiological birth of her placenta, and this will involve some repetition of the key elements.

A calm, unhurried environment will encourage the mother to get to know her baby in her own time and in her own way. She may want to pick the baby up and put it to her breast, or let the baby begin to take in his/her surroundings, and gaze into her eyes. Whilst the term 'bonding' may have become something of a cliché, the concept is vital in promoting a healthy start to parenting. For some women it is important to allow the birth of their placenta to unfold in its own time and to have a sense of completion, relief and triumph, while at the same time changing their focus to the baby:

"How wonderful it is when your placenta comes out because it's all soft and not painful. It's actually quite a feeling of relief because it's all squishy and soft ... it is a really nice feeling."

"I felt it like a first kiss with your favourite boyfriend. That sort of mmm in your belly feeling. That's how it was for me. It was like, ping, big electric thing then I just felt it slide out. It was like wow, and it felt lovely."

For some, the birth of the placenta may be quick and easy, taking minutes, for others it may take a good deal longer. Very occasionally the woman may feel physical discomfort or pain which can be intense and distressing. Some women may still feel overawed by the birth or feel exhausted, cold, shivery, detached or confused, whilst others are keen to 'get it over with', feeling tired and anxious to put the birth of the placenta behind them, to be able to focus on their baby.

4. Actively managed third stage of labour

Active management of the third stage of labour is routinely recommended in nearly all systems of maternity care in high-income countries. It is considered by most doctors and many midwives to be beneficial on a routine basis because research has shown that overall it reduces blood loss and shortens the third stage of labour.

As with many areas of maternity care, there is a bigger picture which should be taken into account, and the issues are not quite as straightforward as many guidelines would seem to suggest. The most recent Cochrane Review (Begley *et al* 2015) suggests that there are benefits and harms associated with active management of the third stage of labour. This review also suggests that we need to consider previous research on this in more detail, and acknowledge its uncertainties, along with its demonstrated harms as well as benefits. This is partly because we have learned that, in healthy women, there is no difference in the chance of excessive bleeding, but there are potential risks and downsides associated with active management. Our experience however, is that changing strongly held beliefs and practices happens only very slowly, especially when these are part of a more medicalised view of birth.

In chapter 5, we discuss the research into this area in depth. In this current chapter, we explain the process and the elements of active management in situations where this is used. This is an important distinction because, as we will explain further below, it is one thing to compare active management to physiological placental birth and another thing to compare the different components of or approaches towards active management of the third stage with each other. There isn't always agreement between different people or areas about the individual components of active management of the third stage and the drugs or medications that are used (WHO 2012). Begley *et al* (2015) emphasise that more research is needed. We will go through the research but will also keep coming back to the fact that there is a great deal of variation in this area (Winter *et al* 2007).

When is active management a good idea?

However a woman plans to birth her placenta, it is important that both she and her midwife and/or doctor should have fully discussed the advantages and disadvantages of the options available and when each may be appropriate. There will be times when active management will be recommended, and a woman who had planned a physiological placental birth may need to revisit her decision if circumstances change and new risk factors develop. We cannot comment on every situation as each is different. Each woman needs to consider factors relating to her pregnancy, how her labour unfolds, her baby (or babies), her general health and any previous labour and birth experiences.

It is always the woman's decision as to whether or not she has drugs or interventions during or after pregnancy and birth and she can decline anything that is offered. As we will discuss further in chapter 5, when a woman is well-nourished, healthy and living in an area where access to emergency medical treatment is readily available, the difference in outcome between options may not vary greatly. But there are situations in which women are deemed to have a greater chance of significant bleeding or may have a greater chance of being compromised if excessive bleeding does occur. Bleeding too much after birth can be very serious indeed and it is helpful for women to know when there may be very good reasons to suggest active management for the birth of the placenta. We have therefore provided some examples of situations in which active management might be a good idea.

The authors of the most recent update of the Cochrane review on this topic point out that: *"Although the studies in the review did not assess women at increased risk of bleeding specifically, it can be deduced from Prendeville's [1988] study that for these women the benefit of reduced blood loss is likely to outweigh the harms. This may lead clinicians to suggest active management of the third stage with a prophylactic uterotonic that contains no ergot, and also deferred cord clamping, though women's choice should always be respected."* (Begley et al 2015).

One question that we often get asked relates to the birth of the placenta following induction of labour. If labour has been induced or augmented (speeded up) using synthetic oxytocin, the woman's ability to produce her own natural oxytocin will be inhibited. This is why any woman who has an oxytocin drip for induction or augmentation of her labour will find that the drip is left up for a while after she has given birth. Turning off the drip too quickly could cause her uterus to relax which may in turn lead to heavy bleeding. For this reason, active management of the third stage will be recommended after any uterotonic drug has been used in labour. In such situations, an additional uterotonic drug is likely to be given to facilitate the birth of the placenta, even when women already have an oxytocin drip in place. In this instance, the drug or medication may be given by intramuscular injection as is usually the case or it may be injected into the intravenous cannula, thereby preventing the need for another injection.

We also know that interventions such as caesarean section and instrumental birth lead to a woman having a higher chance of heavy bleeding. The placenta cannot be born by maternal effort during a caesarean section, but deferred cord clamping (for a minute or so) and cutting is usually possible. There are a number of other situations where active management may be recommended, and we will list some of these below. Having a risk factor doesn't mean that a woman will definitely bleed more than usual, but the chance of this happening may be higher. It is always important to look at this list in relation to the woman's individual circumstances. We don't have good evidence on many of these risk factors, mainly because many of the factors in this list are based on observation, experience or common sense reasoning rather than scientific analysis of the data. These days, there aren't enough women who are considered to be at higher risk of bleeding after birth who have physiological births of their placentas to gather the data we need to help us get a better idea of which of the factors might be implicated with excessive blood loss.

Most obstetric organisations and national maternity bodies (e.g. RCOG 2013, NICE 2017a) have some sort of list of factors which they suggest are linked with a higher chance of excessive bleeding. We have created a list by amalgamating the factors given in a number of these documents, and then added in a few points which may be useful to consider.

Antenatal risk factors for postpartum haemorrhage

- Previous retained placenta or postpartum haemorrhage.
- Maternal haemoglobin level below 85 g/L at the onset of labour (in some areas this is instead expressed as 8.5 g/dL).
- BMI greater than 35 kg/m^2.
- Having had four or more babies (which may be referred to as grand multiparity.
- Bleeding during pregnancy (antepartum haemorrhage).
- Hereditary or pre-existing bleeding disorders.
- Over stretching (overdistention) of the uterus because of multiple pregnancy, excess amniotic fluid (also called polyhydramnios) or having a larger than average baby.
- Having a differently shaped (e.g. bicornuate) uterus.
- Having uterine fibroids.
- Having a low-lying placenta.
- Maternal age 35 or older.

- Asian or African ethnic origin.

Risk factors in labour for postpartum haemorrhage

- Induction of labour.
- Oxytocin use (i.e. to induce or speed up labour).
- Prolonged first, second or third stage of labour.
- Precipitate (very fast) labour.
- Episiotomy.
- Instrumental birth.
- Caesarean section.

Other things to consider

We want to offer a few thoughts about the lists above. We are not suggesting that the factors in the lists might not increase the chance of bleeding after birth, but we don't necessarily know enough about some of them to help individual women decide how they want their placenta to be born. Indeed, many midwives and doctors are uncomfortable with the blanket recommendations found in guidelines. It is always a good idea to talk to a care provider, ask for specific, current evidence and discuss how this relates to your situation and setting. You will then be able to weigh up the advantages and disadvantages within your own individual circumstances. Some things to consider include that:

- Some of the causes of excessive bleeding in a previous birth are linked to something that happened (or was done to the woman) in that birth and they are not likely to occur again in a future birth.
- We cannot accurately predict large babies.
- Where women of particular ethnic origin are identified as being 'at risk' (of anything), this is sometimes because

they are a minority group within a particular area. We also know that women from black and minority ethnic (BAME) groups do not always receive good care, may receive culturally inappropriate care and may not speak English, which can all impact upon their experience and outcomes.

- Midwife Lesley Page carried out some research which challenged the theory that women who have had several babies before have a higher chance of excessive bleeding (Page & McCandlish 2006). This was also confirmed by the work of Briley et al (2014) who noted that, *"although grand multiparity has been associated with PPH, our data reveal multiparity as protective."*
- A placenta that is low-lying early in pregnancy is usually not still low-lying at the time of labour and birth (Heller *et al* 2014).
- When it comes to issues such as maternal size and age, it is difficult to know how much of the 'risk' comes about because of a woman's size and/or age, and how much of the risk is created by the way in which some health professionals treat older and larger women differently, which can lead to over-medicalisation and thus increase their chance of having a problem. It is always important not to focus only on single factors such as age or size but to look at a woman's general health, as this can vary enormously between different women of the same age and/or size.
- The medical definition of prolonged labour varies nationally and internationally and depending on what criteria are used; there is evidence to suggest that, in some areas, women are not being given enough time for the first and second stage of labour, and we do not yet know how this relates to a woman's chance of excessive blood loss during the birth of the placenta.

It is also important to remember that women may have more

than one risk factor and that additional risk factors may develop during labour and/or birth. We don't know how having more than one risk factor impacts on the likelihood of having a postpartum haemorrhage.

What happens in active management of the third stage?

As we have described, there are three components to active management. These are: the giving of a uterotonic drug which makes the woman's uterus contract; the clamping and cutting of the baby's cord; and the removal of the placenta using a technique called controlled cord traction (CCT). However, whether and when these components are used may vary a bit between regions and practitioners.

In previous editions of this book, we noted that there were areas of the world in which it was considered bad practice to give uterotonic drugs before the birth of the placenta. It is possible that this may still be the case in some areas, but recent discussions with colleagues from around the world have led us to believe that most practitioners now agree that a uterotonic drug should be given just after the birth of the baby and before the delivery of the placenta. It is, however, important to establish that a second twin is not present before administering a uterotonic drug. There is also now good evidence (as we described in chapter 3) to defer cord clamping and cutting.

When active management of the third stage is used, the woman is usually asked to adopt a lying down or semi-reclining position as it is then easier for her attendants to apply the different components of active management.

Uterotonic drugs

In most cases, a uterotonic drug is given to the woman by intramuscular (IM) injection, but these drugs are sometimes given in other ways. In a few areas, if a woman has been receiving synthetic oxytocin via an intravenous drip, a separate intramuscular injection may not be given, as explained above. Some of the newer uterotonic drugs are given by mouth, which we will discuss further below. A uterotonic drug can also be given by intravenous injection, but this usually only happens when the woman is having a caesarean section.

Clamping of the cord

When a woman has an actively managed third stage, the cord is clamped and cut, but now that we know that there are benefits to delayed cord clamping, the timing of this has changed in many areas. The current recommendation in areas which practice delayed cord clamping is to give an oxytocic at or immediately after birth while allowing two or three minutes for the baby to transition to extrauterine life and utilise its blood. Two to three minutes after the uterotonic is give, the cord will be clamped and cut. Controlled cord traction will then be used to deliver the placenta. We tend to refer to cord clamping rather than clamping *and* cutting, but both of these tend to occur together.

Usually, the midwife or doctor will place a plastic cord clamp onto the umbilical cord about 3-4cm away from the baby's body. The clamp squeezes the cord and stops the blood flowing between the baby and the placenta, which protects the baby from losing blood when the cord is cut. It is important to avoid pinching the baby's skin or clamping a portion of the baby's gut which may in very rare circumstances protrude into the cord. Another clamp is placed another few centimetres away from the first and nearer the placenta, and scissors are then used to cut the cord in between the clamps.

The plastic clamp stays on the cord after the birth. In some areas, this may be removed after a day or two, but in many places it is left on until the cord drops off, usually between four and ten days after birth. Sometimes, a different kind of clamp, band or tie will be used, but these alternatives are mostly used in out-of-hospital settings and they will have been discussed with (or, more likely, requested by) the woman beforehand. We discuss different options for tying, clamping or burning the cord in chapter 6.

It is common for midwives to offer the woman or her partner the opportunity to cut the cord themselves once the clamps are in place. Indeed, it has almost become a 'rite of passage' for the woman's partner to cut the cord in many countries and even during a caesarean section the cord can be left deliberately long when the baby is born so that the partner can shorten the cord 'ceremonially' once the baby is away from the sterile surgical field.

No matter who cuts the cord, a swab or gloved hand should be held over the cord as it is cut to prevent spillage from the small amount of blood that will remain between the clamp and the place where the cord will be cut. After the cord is cut, the midwife or doctor should double check that the baby's clamp is intact. If a plastic clamp hasn't been used in the first instance (for example if the midwife or doctor used two metal surgical clamps because they were to hand, or at caesarean section), then this will usually be applied sometime after birth and the metal clamp can be removed. This situation may arise if the birth was fast and the relevant equipment had not been gathered or if someone felt a need to separate the baby and mother for newborn life support or resuscitation.

The growth of our knowledge about the value of deferred cord clamping has led to an important advance in some areas, especially in UK hospitals. Some hospitals are now buying equipment which will enable midwives and doctors to give newborn life support or resuscitation help to the baby alongside the woman, so that the cord can remain intact. Before this kind of equipment was developed, the cord was clamped and cut and the baby was taken to a trolley (or resuscitaire) which was often over the other side of the room. In some settings, the resuscitation equipment is in a different room, which many parents find particularly distressing. We understand from colleagues around the world however, that this varies considerably. One Australian colleague told us that she has never seen newborn life support or resuscitation carried out with an intact cord, while in some British hospitals keeping the cord intact is becoming an accepted 'norm' which is promoted and valued amongst health practitioners and parents. A small evaluation of one of the first projects in this area which researched a resuscitation trolley that can be taken to the woman's side found that, *"Immediate stabilisation at birth and resuscitation can be performed successfully and safely at the bedside using this trolley. In most cases this could be achieved with an intact umbilical cord"* (Thomas *et al* 2014). We also note that many community and home birth midwives have for many years performed newborn life support and resuscitation while the cord is still attached.

Controlled cord traction

Controlled cord traction is a specific manoeuvre used to assist the birth of the placenta. It is carried out relatively quickly once there are signs of placental separation. It has long been suggested that it may be advantageous to wait until the cord has lengthened and a fresh trickle of blood has been seen, which indicates that the placenta has separated from the wall of the uterus (Levy & Moore 1985). This practice is known as modified controlled cord traction or modified active management. The midwife or doctor needs to time their actions carefully so that the placenta has separated from the wall of the woman's uterus before controlled cord traction is used. Some uterotonic drugs act within a specific time frame, so it should not be delayed once separation has occurred.

The practitioner will sometimes place their hand on the mother's abdomen so that they can feel when the woman has a contraction of her uterus. A container might be placed between the woman's legs to catch and assess blood loss as the midwife or doctor delivers the placenta. The midwife or doctor then uses gentle, firm sustained traction (pulling) on the cord whilst 'guarding' (supporting) the woman's uterus with their other hand. This guarding ensures that the woman's uterus does not become inverted (turned inside out) during the procedure.

Prophylaxis or treatment?

There are two different ways of using the components of active management of the birth of the placenta. The first is as a specific treatment for excessive bleeding. Uterotonic drugs are effective in stopping excessive bleeding in most cases; they undoubtedly have saved the lives of many women and will continue to do so. Excessive bleeding can happen whether or not the woman experiences a physiological placental birth or an actively managed third stage. But it is important to note that, if a woman decides to have a physiological birth of her placenta and experiences excessive bleeding during or after this, uterotonic drugs can still be used as a treatment. We do not know enough about whether using a uterotonic drug as a treatment is as effective as using prophylactic active management.

The second way of using active management of the third stage of labour is as a preventative measure (or prophylaxis). In chapter 5, we will discuss the research which compares the two approaches of expectant management and active management of the third stage. The research that we discuss here looks at the use of these drugs as an element of active management; that is, as prophylaxis rather than treatment.

However, we would like to add one important note. In a study carried in New Zealand, Dixon *et al* (2013) noted that uterotonic drugs seemed to be twice as effective as a treatment for excessive bleeding in the healthy women who initially chose to have physiological placental birth than in the healthy women who had planned active management. So it is not only reasonable for a healthy women who has experienced a physiological labour and birth to opt for a physiological placental birth, but it may be that, if she needs drug treatment, this will be more effective than if she had chosen intervention in the first place.

In the remainder of this chapter, we will look at each of the components of active management (uterotonic drugs, cord clamping and controlled cord traction) in more depth before discussing how long active management takes.

Uterotonic drugs

Uterotonic drugs are powerful substances which cause the woman's uterus to contract. There are several different kinds and they may be used at a number of different points during and after labour. Uterotonic drugs may be used after the baby is born, either during the third stage of labour itself or occasionally in the postnatal (after birth) period if a woman experiences a secondary postpartum haemorrhage. Some of the drugs that we will discuss in this section are also used for inducing labour (see Wickham 2018a) or to speed labour up if it is perceived to be progressing too slowly.

Drugs used to prevent or treat heavy bleeding

Over the past few decades, until fairly recently, the most commonly used uterotonic drug was a synthetic form of oxytocin known by the brand names of Syntocinon or Pitocin.

Synthetic oxytocin works by causing the uterus to contract and it is usually given as an IM injection. Sometimes it is given intravenously (IV). Common but easily treatable short-term side effects of oxytocin include headache, the woman's heart rate slowing or becoming irregular and lower blood pressure. Rarely, problems such as an allergic reaction can occur. Synthetic oxytocin is known to interfere with a woman's production of her own oxytocin and it can cause maternal depression and anxiety (Kroll-Desrosiers *et al* 2017), interfere with breastfeeding, and affect a woman's subsequent birth experiences (Buckley 2011, 2015). Such consequences are often not measured in research studies, which tend to focus on short-term outcomes. Oxytocin is sometimes combined with another drug called ergometrine (or Ergonovine). So let's look at that next before discussing how they are used together.

Ergometrine is also given by IM injection but where oxytocin works on the oxytocin receptors in the uterus, ergometrine causes the uterus to contract by working directly on smooth muscle, which includes the uterus. The effect of ergometrine lasts for longer than oxytocin; up to three hours. The common side effects of ergometrine include changes in blood pressure, headache, nausea and vomiting. Ergometrine is also known to be transferred to the baby through breastmilk and drug information leaflets state that women should be told of this, but we are aware that this doesn't often happen in practice. Research evidence shows that women who have ergometrine during the third stage of labour breastfed for a shorter period of time (Begley 1990b, Jordan *et al* 2009, Buckley 2011).

The most common version of the combined form of oxytocin and ergometrine is called Syntometrine. A 1ml vial of Syntometrine is made up of 5 mg of oxytocin and 0.5mg of ergometrine. In recent years, however, the combined medication has become less popular, and there has been a trend towards using Syntocinon on its own rather than in combination with ergometrine (NICE 2007, 2017a). This is because of the potential side effects of ergometrine, particularly nausea and vomiting and raised blood pressure. The raising of women's blood pressure is of significant concern and ergometrine is not used in women who have high blood pressure or related problems. Even when the combined form was in common use, practitioners tended to use oxytocin on its own for women whose blood pressure was of concern.

Over the past few years, researchers have also been examining the use of other drugs in active management of the birth of the placenta. Much attention has been given to a class of drugs called synthetic prostaglandins, and the most common of these is called misoprostol (known in the USA as Cytotec). Misoprostol is a synthetic prostaglandin analogue originally developed to treat stomach ulcers but found to stimulate the uterus. This can be given by a number of routes, including orally (by mouth), sublingually (under the tongue) or into the woman's vagina or rectum and the time that it takes to work depends on how it is given. Much of the research attention is now focusing on giving misoprostol by mouth, but it is also worth knowing that, sometimes, fast acting forms of synthetic prostaglandin may be given in an emergency situation, i.e. to treat a postpartum haemorrhage.

Misoprostol works on the prostaglandin receptors and common side effects include abdominal pain, headache, diarrhoea, dizziness, nausea, vomiting and developing a rash. Rare but more serious side effects include excessive bleeding, raised temperature and uterine hyperstimulation. Unlike oxytocin, misoprostol does not need to be kept in a cool, dark place, which is a potential advantage, particularly in hot countries and especially where refrigeration is not available.

Another drug which is becoming more widely used in this aspect of care is carbetocin (also known as Duratocin). Carbetocin has an action similar to oxytocin, in that it binds to oxytocin receptors. Because carbetocin is a relatively new drug, we have less knowledge about its side effects and their frequency. We do know that carbetocin should not be used in women with asthma or heart disease. We also know that it can have long-term effects on a woman's reproduction and mothering (in the same way that oxytocin affects this), but we do not know nearly enough about this (Buckley 2015).

The crucial difference between oxytocin and carbetocin is that carbetocin has been developed to be longer acting. The effects of oxytocin only last for a few minutes, and the longer acting carbetocin is often preferred by obstetricians when women have a caesarean section. Some obstetricians feel that women who have had an anaesthetic and major surgery may be less likely to notice if they are bleeding too much afterwards, and prefer carbetocin in this situation.

Like misoprostol, carbetocin can be made in a heat-stable form (Rosales-Ortiz *et al* 2014) which does not need to be kept in a fridge. It is thus a better option where refrigeration is not easily available. Many people interpret this as being specifically useful in countries that are hot and resource-poor, but it is also an issue in some settings in high-income countries. Midwives working in rural areas, for instance, can sometimes be on the road for hours at a time and heat-stable uterotonic drugs are a significant advantage in such situations.

Early research in this area suggested that intramuscular carbetocin may be as effective as intramuscular oxytocin and it appears that carbetocin has fewer side effects in the women who receive it (Leung *et al* 2006, Su *et al* 2009). The research into this drug continues to be promising, as we will discuss further below.

Finally, a drug called tranexamic acid is also being considered and researched for use in active management of the third stage. Tranexamic acid is actually not a uterotonic drug but it reduces blood loss (by causing blood clotting, which can be a problem as well as an advantage). It is sometimes prescribed for women who have heavy periods as well as being used during surgical procedures. To our knowledge, it is not being used instead of a uterotonic drug in active management of the third stage of labour, but in combination with uterotonics in a few research studies around the world.

A Cochrane review looked at tranexamic acid (TA) and concluded that, when used in addition to uterotonic medications, it *"decreases postpartum blood loss and prevents PPH and blood transfusions following vaginal birth and* [caesarean section] *in women at low risk of PPH based on studies of mixed quality. There is insufficient evidence to draw conclusions about serious side effects, but there is an increase in the incidence of minor side effects with the use of TA. Effects of TA on thromboembolic events and mortality as well as its use in high-risk women should be investigated further."* (Novikova *et al* 2015). We are not going to look further at tranexamic acid, because it is not in common use and isn't one of the uterotonic drugs compared in the research on this topic, but we wanted to offer a brief explanation as some people will encounter this drug, possibly as part of a research trial.

There are a few other things that we want to mention which apply to all uterotonic drugs. In some situations, the woman and her midwife find themselves in a race against the clock to birth the placenta before the woman's cervix begins to close again as a result of the drugs used. Of course, although the word 'close' is commonly used in this context, the cervix is never completely closed. Menstrual blood can get out, and sperm can get in. But it is possible for the opening of the cervix to be too narrow for the placenta to pass though. This can lead to the woman being diagnosed as having a retained placenta, for which surgery is usually offered. Retained placenta is another important outcome measure when researchers evaluate the drugs used in active management, and we will return to this point. It is also important to know that retained placenta can happen when the placenta hasn't separated from the wall of the uterus.

We will also look at the rate of bleeding when women have different types of placental birth, and a key thing to remember here is that uterotonic drugs do not prevent all cases of excessive bleeding. This is because there are other reasons for bleeding after birth and/or during the birth of the placenta. For instance, a woman may bleed from a tear or an episiotomy, and certain blood clotting disorders can also cause bleeding to be excessive. None of these are treatable by the use of uterotonic drugs. Excessive bleeding can happen during a caesarean section, and this is often treated by tranexamic acid. In theory, excessive bleeding from a tear or episiotomy could be treated with tranexamic acid, although this is unlikely to happen in practice as the fastest and most effective way of treating this is to apply local pressure and to suture (or stitch) the wound, which most midwives and doctors can do very quickly when this is occasionally necessary.

Sometimes, parents ask whether drugs contain animal products or are suitable for those who have allergies or follow religious food laws. One of us (Sara) has addressed this in a related book, and the answer is the same. The drugs that are mentioned as being used in induction of labour in the quote below are the same (uterotonic) drugs that are used in active management of the birth of the placenta.

"Many countries do not require pharmaceutical companies to label drugs in the way that food production companies label foods. In many countries, inactive ingredients aren't listed at all. Sometimes, an ingredient can be made from one of several sources. The company may change this, they are under no obligation to label drugs and it may not even be possible to find out what a particular batch of a drug contains from company records. This is particularly the case when drugs are manufactured in countries such as China.

Drugs and medicines do come with product information sheets, and these will contain general information about what the drug contains. They will also contain information about the risks and side effects of the drug. You may be able to get copies of this sheet from your midwife or doctor, and often they are also available online.

Drugs which mimic or contain hormones (including some of those used in induction, contraception and menopause treatment) are often animal derived. This may be the case even if they are described as synthetic.

If you are very keen to find out about a drug and cannot get the information you need from the label, you may wish to contact a local pharmacist (perhaps via the hospital, as most hospitals have pharmacy departments) or the pharmaceutical company directly. This may or may not help you get the information you are seeking, but it is worth a try." (Wickham 2018a).

Finally, although it is very rare, there is always a small risk in having any drug because medicines and injections can be mixed up, and human factors are an important consideration. Jean Robinson noted this in the foreword to an earlier version of this book:

"When randomised trials report on outcome from any extra intervention, they do not mention the additional risks each one brings. With every drug comes a risk that it will be given to the wrong person in the wrong dose or at the wrong time. And drugs given by injection are riskier than those given orally, since their diverse effects are likely to be more severe, and they can be injected into the wrong place as well as the wrong person. For additional procedures, each new intake of staff has to practise and learn on someone - like the mother whose cord was broken when the medical student was told to practise controlled cord traction.

Those of us who often dip into medical literature, soon realise that adverse effects of intervention often surface only when a different treatment becomes available for comparison. Proponents or producers of the new drug or treatment will then happily write about the disadvantages of the old, in order to convert colleagues to the new. This is also true of different oxytocic drugs used to reduce haemorrhage risk in the third stage." (Robinson 1999: 8)

Although rare, we know of one case where neonatal convulsions were caused in a baby given an oxytocic drug instead of Vitamin K, and another where a baby died when a mother was given Syntometrine instead of pethidine when she was in labour. It is always a good idea to ask what drug you are being given, for lots of reasons, rather than to unquestioningly allow health professionals to give you or your baby an injection.

Evidence of effectiveness and safety

In 2018, a Cochrane review (Gallos *et al* 2018) offered some very helpful information on the effectiveness and safety of different kinds of uterotonic drugs. Prior to the publication of this review, we had had to gather information from a variety of sources for this section of the book, but the review included data from 140 randomised controlled trials which had involved 88,947 women. There are a few issues (as is always the case with research) that we want to highlight before we discuss the findings and the conclusions that the authors reached about the effectiveness and safety of the different uterotonic drugs, but we are confident that this review is a good basis for our discussion of this topic, as the authors have analysed a large number of studies in order to compare the different drugs.

The first issue that we want to briefly mention is that the trials in the Gallos *et al* (2018) review were mostly carried out in hospital settings. This means that we don't know whether the situation would be different in out-of-hospital settings such as midwifery-led units and when women birth at home. They also predominantly focus on the experiences of women who gave birth at or after 37 weeks of gestation, so we can't know if things are different for women who birth before this.

Many of the trials were deemed to be at *"uncertain risk of bias"* (Gallos *et al* 2018), which means the review authors were unsure about how good the design of the research was. Often, this was because the original researchers didn't give enough detail. This type of potential bias isn't uncommon. It is helpful that the authors of the Cochrane review have shared their assessment that this problem *"...primarily impacted on our confidence in comparisons involving carbetocin trials more than other uterotonics."* (Gallos *et al* 2018).

The results of this review were a bit surprising to some people. The key conclusion in relation to effectiveness was that, *"...ergometrine plus oxytocin, misoprostol plus oxytocin, and carbetocin were more effective drugs for reducing excessive bleeding at childbirth than oxytocin which is the current standard drug used to prevent this condition."* (Gallos *et al* 2018). So even though there has been a movement towards using oxytocin on its own, as recommended by the WHO (2012), this may change again. Gallos *et al* (2018) have shown that, actually, oxytocin on its own may not be as effective as (1) the more traditional combination of ergometrine plus oxytocin (often known as Syntometrine), (2) misoprostol plus oxytocin, a newer combination and then (3) carbetocin. One issue with carbetocin, however, is this: *"Carbetocin has the least side-effects among the top three drug options, but to date studies of carbetocin were small and of poor quality."* (Gallos *et al* 2018). So future studies involving larger numbers of women may change these results.

These studies and more potential changes are not as far off as one might think. Gallos *et al* (2018) specifically mentioned two large, ongoing studies which are nearing completion. One of these is comparing several different regimes, one of which is carbetocin. The other, which set out to compare carbetocin to oxytocin, was published just before this book went to press. Widmer *et al* (2018) randomised 29,645 women across 23 sites in ten countries. They focused on healthy women who were pregnant with a single baby and expected to give birth vaginally. The women received either 100 μg of heat-stable carbetocin or 10IU of oxytocin. The management of the third stage was carried out according to WHO (2012) guidelines. Blood loss was measured for the first hour, or for two hours after birth if it continued.

This particular study was a non-inferiority trial; a type of study carried out when the existing treatment is thought or known to be beneficial and it is deemed unethical to use a new treatment and a placebo. The idea is to see whether the new drug (in this case, carbetocin) is as good as (or non-inferior to) the existing one. The double negatives can be confusing, but it is done in the name of ethics. The authors found that, *"Heat-stable carbetocin was noninferior to oxytocin for the prevention of blood loss of at least 500 ml or the use of additional uterotonic agents. Noninferiority was not shown for the outcome of blood loss of at least 1000 ml; low event rates for this outcome reduced the power of the trial."* (Widmer *et al* 2018).

Currently, there is considerable variation in practice in different areas, and this is unsurprising given the state of flux of the research on this topic. In just a few years, there has been a widespread change in the favoured drug and several studies have been carried out around the world. It is really helpful to look at reviews such as that by Gallos *et al* (2018) in order to gather together and compare the results of many different studies, and it is equally useful to consider new studies like Widmer *et al* (2018) in order to consider in what direction things might move in the future. But, in reality, the drugs and protocols used in a hospital or region are often influenced just as much or more by the preferences of local practitioners. It is not uncommon for a hospital which carried out a trial to continue favouring the practice or the drug which seemed to be the most effective in its trial, even if the weight of the evidence swings towards another option being better. This is another reminder that evidence is interpreted by humans and isn't always as objective as we might think.

In common with much of the research into this area, the studies included in this review used quantitative measures of maternal wellbeing, with the main one of these being blood loss. As we will discuss in the next chapter, there are wider issues to be considered, and the reviewers add these thoughts:

"Consultation with our consumer group has

demonstrated a need for more research into PPH outcomes identified as priorities for women and their families, such as women's views regarding the drugs used, clinical signs of excessive blood loss, neonatal unit admissions and breastfeeding at discharge. Trials to date have rarely investigated these outcomes. Consumers also considered the side-effects of uterotonic drugs to be important and these were often not reported. A set of standardised PPH outcomes are being developed and will be incorporated in future updates of this review. We would hope that future trials would also consider adopting those outcomes. Finally, future systematic reviews could compare the effects of different doses and ways of administering the most effective drugs." (Gallos *et al* 2018).

Cord clamping

As we described in chapter 2, the medical approach to birth which developed in the 1600s led to the widespread practice of immediate cord clamping (Muza 2017). However, *"…early cord clamping had no specific rationale, and it probably entered the protocol by default because it was already part of standard practice. When this package was shown to reduce postpartum haemorrhage in the 1980s early cord clamping became enshrined in the modern management of labour"* (Weeks 2007: 312).

Nowadays, we know that there are significant advantages to leaving the cord intact while the baby makes its transition to life outside the womb (Mercer & Erickson-Owens 2010, 2014, Hutchon 2012, WHO 2012, Bhatt *et al* 2013, McDonald *et al* 2013, Hooper *et al* 2015). As a result, there is an increasing trend to avoid clamping and cutting the cord immediately after the baby's birth, even when women have active management of the birth of their placenta. In this section, we will not be reiterating the benefits of deferred cord clamping, which we have already covered, but we will look at how this relates to active management of the third stage of labour.

We also noted that both the National Institute of Health and Clinical Excellence (NICE 2017a, 2017b) and the World Health Organization (WHO 2017) recommend that a baby's cord should not be clamped within the first one to three minutes following birth. The WHO (2017) also recommends that, where women opt for active management of the third stage of labour, this should incorporate delayed cord clamping so as to enable the baby's blood from the placenta to move into the baby's body, which we know reduces the likelihood of anaemia (Begley *et al* 2015). There is variation in how this is interpreted and a lack of evidence to guide practice (RCOG 2015). We know of many areas where a uterotonic is still given with the birth of the baby's shoulder, and other areas where this seems to be changing. A midwife in one English hospital, for instance, told us that, *"...in practice what is now happening is that Syntocinon is given once the baby is born, the cord is left to pulsate – sometimes until it stops – and then clamped/cut and controlled cord traction or maternal effort is used to birth the placenta."*

There is also some debate about whether the baby needs to be in a particular position relative to the placenta. A number of national guidelines make recommendations about this, but without citing evidence. The authors of a Cochrane review (McDonald *et al* 2013) clearly state that: *"Palethorpe (2010) and colleagues sought to evaluate studies related to the effects for mother and baby of alternative positions for the baby between birth and cord clamping to assess the influence of gravity on placental transfusion. However, no randomised controlled trials were identified for comparison and they concluded there was a need for large, well designed randomised controlled trials to be undertaken to ascertain what effect gravity may have on placental transfusion at vaginal and caesarean births related to short- and longer-term outcomes for mothers and babies."*

In 2014, researchers from Argentina (Vain *et al* 2014)

looked at 391 normally-born, vigorous newborn babies who were held either at the level of the mother's vagina or on her abdomen or chest just after birth. The babies were weighed immediately after birth and then again after their cord had been clamped. The researchers then looked for any differences in the two weight measurements, which acted as a measure of the volume of blood that was transferred to the baby from the placenta. There was no difference between the two groups of babies in this respect (Vain *et al* 2014).

In a linked commentary in *The Lancet*, Raju (2014) noted that the introduction of delayed cord clamping into practice has been sporadic. He suggests that one reason for this is the logistical problem of practitioners feeling they need to hold babies at the level of the introitus until their cords have been cut. At this point in the birth of a new family, he explained, pretty much everybody else in the room, including the baby, wants the baby to be skin to skin with its mother.

It is hard to know whether or not the gravity question is playing a significant part in this, but Raju's concern about the implementation of deferred cord clamping was echoed by the findings of a recent survey by the Positive Birth Movement, which found that: *"...whilst over 90%* [of parents who responded] *were aware of the benefits of Optimal Cord Clamping (OCC), and 75% specifically requested it either in their birth plan or during labour, 40% of parents reported that their babies did not receive OCC, with an alarming 31% stating that their baby's cord was clamped in less than a minute. One fifth of respondents stated the cord was cut immediately."* (Positive Birth Movement 2018). The results of this survey may not be representative of all parents' experiences, as the sample was self-selected and may include more parents who had an experience which led them to want to share their views, but it is still deeply worrying that parents are not having their wishes respected. There does seem to be a lot of variation in guidelines and between systems, countries, hospitals and practitioners.

Another related issue concerns a practice called 'cord

milking'. It is possible that cord milking derived from the discomfort that more technocratically-minded practitioners feel about waiting for a minute or three before clamping and cutting the cord. At some point, somebody came up with the notion that, if the practitioner used their hand to 'milk' or 'strip' the cord, thus pushing the blood from the placenta towards the baby, they might get the same amount of blood transfer without having to wait before clamping and cutting the cord. Currently, the bottom line on cord milking in the guidelines that we have seen is that there isn't enough evidence to know whether this is beneficial, and so it is not currently recommended (McDonald *et al* 2013, RCOG 2015).

Finally, people often ask whether deferred cord clamping is incompatible with the taking of the baby's blood from the cord. The answer is no. No matter whether blood is being taken for a screening test (such as to measure blood gases or the baby's iron levels, determine the baby's blood group or find out if the baby is rhesus positive or rhesus negative) or in relation to cord blood banking, this should not interfere with deferred cord clamping. Some women have reported that cord blood banking has reduced their options and negatively interfered with the time that they would have had together as a family immediately after birth. If cord blood banking is something that you are considering or asked about, we would urge you to do lots of research before making a decision.

Controlled cord traction

For many years, and until very recently, controlled cord traction was believed to be an important part of the package of active management of the third stage of labour. It is applied after an oxytocic drug has caused a strong uterine contraction following the baby's birth, and once the placenta appears to have separated from the woman's uterine wall.

However, the Cochrane review (Begley *et al* 2015) on third stage management suggests that we do not know for sure whether controlled cord traction actually contributes to reducing blood loss at birth. It may, Begley *et al* (2015) argue, even increase the likelihood of secondary bleeding (bleeding at a later stage) after birth.

In fact, the story of controlled cord traction is a good example of an obstetric tale that is far more common than many people realise. An intervention or practice is introduced because it is thought to be a good idea. Often this is based on the notion that women need help during birth, and sometimes profits can be made from selling the idea or the means of implementing it. In time, the practice becomes common and, often, a point is reached where anyone who doesn't follow it is considered to be unsafe or not up-to-date. The fact that it was only based on an idea has been forgotten, and it has now become the norm against which other practices need to be measured. In such circumstances it is now nature and physiology that are doubted, and have to prove themselves against this unscientifically proven and possibly economically-driven practice that someone once thought was a good idea.

We know that controlled cord traction can cause problems, and a small number of women find this procedure painful or uncomfortable, especially if it is carried out too early, before the placenta is separating. As we have already mentioned, there is a rare chance that the midwife or doctor may cause the uterus to invert, and this is why the procedure involves using a hand to 'guard' or support the woman's uterus. Uterine inversion can still happen even when precautions are used, although this is extremely rare.

Other potential downsides include the risk of pulling out a placenta that has not yet completely separated or that is attached to the uterus in a way that could lead to significant bleeding. However, if the placenta is attached in a way that is problematic, it may need to be surgically removed no matter what decision the women had made about the birth of her placenta. When someone uses controlled cord traction, there is a chance that the cord may snap or be pulled off at the point where it connects to the placenta. This is also unusual, but it does happen and, if the practitioner cannot reach the end of the cord then a manual removal of the placenta with a regional anaesthetic might be considered necessary.

All of the above things can happen when the placenta is completely healthy and normal. However, occasionally the placenta grows with an extra lobe or the cord is attached right on the edge of the placenta. In both of these situations, controlled cord traction may be more likely to cause a problem than if the placenta is allowed to birth naturally. We are aware of situations where midwives have been very glad that a woman chose to have a physiological placental birth because the cord and/or placenta was fragile and may not have remained intact if controlled cord traction had been used. For these reasons, it is not a good idea to fiddle with or pull on the cord when the birth of the placenta is physiological. In fact, any handling of the uterus can cause pain and bleeding so, unless there is a need to manually help the woman's uterus to contract in order to manage bleeding, so-called 'fundal fiddling' should also be avoided.

The routine practice of controlled cord traction was challenged in 2012, when an important study was published. Gülmezoglu *et al* (2012) carried out a multicentre randomised controlled trial in 16 hospitals and two health care centres in Argentina, Egypt, India, Kenya, the Philippines, South Africa, Thailand and Uganda. These countries are all in parts of the world where postpartum haemorrhage is a significant cause of severe illness and maternal death. One of the reasons for this study was to see whether the training of birth attendants in such countries needed to include controlled cord traction or could focus solely on the use of oxytocin.

The idea of Gülmezoglu *et al*'s (2012) study was to see whether the controlled cord traction component of active management could be omitted without increasing the chance of severe bleeding. Women who were expecting single babies were randomly allocated to receive either a 'simplified' package (which meant they would have synthetic oxytocin but would deliver their placenta with the help of gravity and maternal effort) or the 'full package' of synthetic oxytocin, cord clamping (at between 1 and 3 minutes) and controlled cord traction. About 11,800 women were in each group.

The results showed that controlled cord traction had very little effect on the risk of severe bleeding and Gülmezoglu *et al* (2012) concluded that, *"…haemorrhage prevention programmes for non-hospital settings can safely focus on use of oxytocin."*

A later Cochrane review (Hofmeyr *et al* 2015) of the value of controlled cord traction included two other (much smaller) studies. The reviewers were considering whether controlled cord traction was of use in settings where highly trained midwives and doctors can deal with the consequences of a problem. Gülmezoglu *et al* (2012) were considering settings in which educators feel they need to carefully choose key messages and focus on teaching the things that can really make a difference.

The results were that, *"CCT has the advantage of reducing the risk of manual removal of the placenta in some circumstances, and evidence suggests that CCT can be routinely offered during the third stage of labour, provided the birth attendant has the necessary skills. CCT should remain a core competence of skilled birth attendants. However, the limited benefits of CCT in terms of severe PPH would not justify the major investment which would be needed to provide training in CCT skills for birth attendants who do not have formal training. Women who prefer a less interventional approach to management of the third stage of labour can be reassured that when a uterotonic agent is used, routine use of CCT can be omitted from the 'active management' package without increased risk of severe PPH, but that the risk of manual removal of the placenta may be increased."* (Hofmeyr *et al* 2015).

So although controlled cord traction is still in routine use in many areas where active management of the third stage is used, any woman who wishes to have active management of the third stage of her labour but who does not like the idea of controlled cord traction may wish to consider this Cochrane review.

How long does active management take?

Typically, an actively managed third stage will take between five to ten minutes after the baby is born. When uterotonic drugs containing ergot are given it is usually assumed that the placenta needs to be birthed within a relatively short length of time, and before the circular muscles around the cervix contract. In areas where Syntocinon is used, there may be less of a sense of urgency. We do know that women who have active management of the third stage of labour are more likely to bleed if there is a delay in the placenta being born (Begley et al 2015). A common scenario is that the oxytocic drug is given either during the birth or as soon as the baby is born, and the cord is clamped and cut after two or three minutes. The midwife or doctor will then watch for signs of placental separation and, as soon as these are seen, they will apply controlled cord traction and pull the placenta out. If the placenta doesn't come the first time, the midwife or doctor may wait for two or three minutes before trying again.

The shorter duration of an actively managed third stage is often cited as an advantage of this approach. However, some women who birth their placentas physiologically do so very quickly too. It is also important to remember that waiting for a placenta to be born is not like other kinds of waiting. The woman and family have a new baby to meet, greet and cuddle. It is the rare woman who is frustrated at having to wait for a shower just because her placenta hasn't been born. In hospitals, waiting for the placenta can also give the new family a bit of much-needed breathing space, as other things have to wait until this has happened, which allows time for skin to skin cuddling and the oxytocin-filled bonding of the new family. It is important to remember, however, that if a woman has had an episiotomy or has sustained a significant tear during the birth, earlier examination and repair of the tear or episiotomy is advantageous as earlier suturing is associated with less bruising and bleeding.

Manual removal of the placenta

We mentioned in the previous chapter that women who aim for a physiological placental birth may be advised to have active management if there is a problem, and that there are also situations in which manual removal of the placenta is recommended. Manual removal may also be recommended in some situations where women opt for active management but the placenta does not come out easily.

In the UK, NICE (2014) guidance suggests that the third stage should be considered delayed if it takes longer than half an hour to deliver the placenta by active management. In cases where the placenta does not come out (retained placenta) following active or physiological management, the woman will usually be told that the placenta needs to be manually removed. This procedure involves a doctor putting their hand inside the woman's uterus to remove the placenta. This would be very painful without anaesthetic and so, in high-income countries, an epidural, spinal or general anaesthesia will be offered.

It is very important that a woman gives her informed consent to manual removal of the placenta and that no attempt to manually remove her placenta is made before the anaesthetic is fully effective. Women have sometimes been told by an obstetrician that her placenta may be 'just inside' or behind her cervix and that they can try to remove it without the need to move to an operating theatre where the woman will be attended by a surgical team and given an anaesthetic. This is not considered good practice and, if manual removal of the placenta is needed, the woman should have effective pain relief. Appropriate manual removal also entails a thorough examination of the woman's uterus to ensure that all the placenta will be removed, reducing the chance of a later infection or haemorrhage.

Manual removal of the placenta does carry risks, like any other surgical procedure, even when done under optimal conditions. Common risks include infection, not fully removing the placenta and intrauterine adhesions, or internal scar tissue. Less common but serious risks include perforating the woman's uterus or causing damage to the woman's cervix or birth canal. These possible risks would require immediate emergency treatment. This is another reason that, where facilities are available, many practitioners believe that manual removal should only be carried out in an operating theatre. If manual removal is offered, the woman should be told of all possible risks and benefits. Although any procedure at this point interferes with the time that a woman and her family has to bond with their baby immediately after birth, sometimes treatment is essential. For this reason, it can be very useful for women to think ahead of time about what they would want to happen if at any stage something happened which meant they might need to move to 'plan B' or even 'plan C' (please see Wickham 2018b for more on this).

It is important to know that delaying manual removal often leads to the spontaneous delivery of the placenta (Cronk & Flint 1989, Urner *et al* 2014). Although it is not common practice in maternity care systems to take a 'wait and see' approach following a managed third stage which has not resulted in the birth of the placenta after about 30 minutes, we know of quite a few cases where women who were scheduled to have their placenta removed under anaesthetic have managed to push their placentas out once the effect of the uterotonic drugs has worn off. Unless the woman is bleeding heavily, as with all other aspects of pregnancy and birth, a woman who is offered manual removal of her placenta may wish to think about the pros and cons of this and ask whether this needs to be carried out immediately or whether waiting for a while is an option.

5. Third stage research trials

Active management of the third stage of labour, like many other birth interventions, was introduced without research which considered its full impact on the mother and baby. Over the last decades, a growing number of researchers, practitioners and parents have questioned whether active management of the third stage of labour should be a routine practice. We haven't included discussion of every single study in here, as that would make the book far too long, so we have picked some key landmarks to illustrate the development of our knowledge in this area.

There are a few important things to note. Within the medical literature, there is little discussion of 'the birth of the placenta'; most of the research and discussion focuses on 'the third stage of labour'. This emphasis reflects the importance that has been placed on viewing labour and birth as a set of discrete and measurable stages which can and should be obstetrically observed and managed. Such an approach fails to appreciate the active involvement of the birthing woman or the variation of the normal rhythms of the journey. As we will show in this chapter however, this situation is changing.

The research in this area is also limited in that it focuses on a narrow range of short-term physical outcomes rather than taking a more holistic approach. The effects of uterotonic drugs and the other possible harms of active management should also be given more consideration (Begley *et al* 2015) as we discussed in chapter 4.

Another issue that we want to raise about the studies generally is that most of the women in the studies discussed below gave birth in hospital, where the birth of both the baby and the placenta is usually medically managed. This setting and approach will not necessarily provide the kind of environment conducive to the flow of birth hormones that are needed to help the placenta to be born. This raises a number of questions about the validity of the outcomes reported for physiological birth of the placenta. A key criticism of the randomised controlled trials which have been carried out to date is that, in all groups in the trials, the third stage is in fact 'managed.' Odent (2002, 1998b), Fahy (2009) and others also suggest that expectant third stage management is defined in negative terms in relation to active management, rather than in positive terms and in relation to factors that may promote the safety and efficiency of a physiological placental birth. They and others believe that the research is therefore biased towards managed third stage from the outset and that disturbances to the physiological processes have a major influence on the third stage. They claim that, in the randomised trials to date, physiological processes are *"highly disturbed both in the study groups and the control groups"* (Odent 1998b).

We would argue that, because of this, it may be helpful to think about three rather than two approaches to the birth of the placenta. The most medical of these would be active management of the third stage, which we discussed in chapter 4. The most holistic would be physiological birth of the placenta. This is where a woman is able to birth her placenta in a relaxed way, in a woman-centred environment which is conducive to physiological birth, without intervention (unless this becomes necessary because a problem is experienced).

The third approach – which is somewhere in between – is sometimes called physiological birth of the placenta but would more accurately be defined as 'expectant management of the third stage of labour.' This term is used in many of the research trials that we discuss in the following pages and better describes what happens when active management is not used in a hospital setting within an obstetric paradigm. It is important to mention this because most of these studies don't compare active management with physiological placental birth; they compare active management with expectant management. This is not to say that physiological birth of the placenta cannot occur within a hospital setting.

The main difference is not in place but ideology. Good research which reflects more holistic ideology takes into account women's individual health, and environment.

The question of normal blood loss

Another important issue that we need to discuss in depth before we detail the individual studies is the question of blood loss and of some of the definitions that midwifery and medical practitioners use to describe women's experiences of this. It is normal for women to bleed to some extent after they have a baby and this is the usual response to having given birth. The question of what amount of blood loss is normal is an important one, both in practice and in research. We know that there is wide variation in the amount of blood loss and the length of time for which women bleed (Marchant *et al* 1999). But if blood loss is excessive or if the woman does not feel well, urgent help is required.

Excessive bleeding is most likely to occur within the first 24 hours after birth and this is called a primary postpartum haemorrhage. Many obstetric and midwifery textbooks cite the 'four Ts' as being the causes of primary postpartum haemorrhage. These are tone (the uterus is not well contracted), trauma (the woman has a tear or injury to an area such as her perineum, vagina or uterus, which is bleeding), tissue (a piece of the placenta and/or membranes has remained in the woman's uterus or cervix, which may be preventing it from contracting) and thrombin (which describes a problem in the woman's blood clotting mechanisms). If excessive bleeding occurs after 24 hours but before 6 weeks after birth, this is called a secondary postpartum haemorrhage.

As we noted above, postpartum haemorrhage which occurs after the birth of the placenta can be caused when part of the placenta remains behind after birth. This is one reason why midwives and doctors check the placenta after it has been born. If part of the placenta remains in the uterus, it can cause infection and secondary postpartum haemorrhage and doctors will often recommend that the retained part of the placenta is removed. This usually entails a surgical procedure which involves a doctor dilating the woman's cervix and using sterile instruments to remove the part of the placenta that has remained in the woman's uterus.

Both practitioners and researchers commonly define the cut-off point between normal blood loss and postpartum haemorrhage to be 500ml. This does not account for individuals' responses to blood loss, which vary significantly. One of us (Sara) regularly speaks to large groups of midwives about placental birth, with the following experience:

"I often ask the midwives present to put up their hands if they have seen a woman lose more than 500mls of blood and be fine. Almost everybody raises their hands. Then I ask them if they have seen a woman lose more than 1000mls and be fine; again, almost all the hands go up, and finally I ask if they have seen a woman lose less than 500mls of blood and be compromised. Quite a few midwives raise their hands at this point too. We have to understand that the measurement of blood loss alone is not helpful. We also need to look at how the woman copes with that blood loss on physical and other levels, and base decisions about transfer (in the case of a home or other out-of-hospital birth) and treatment on the basis of how the woman is rather than on an arbitrary and often inaccurate measurement of how much she bleeds." (Edwards & Wickham 2011:56).

If blood loss causes ill health in the mother, this is detrimental to both mother and child. As the above quote shows, this may occur even in the absence of a large bleed, and if women are not feeling well then they should ensure that they get appropriate attention whether or not their blood loss was considered 'normal'.

There has been a growing tendency towards redefining the definition of normal blood loss. Bloomfield and Gordon (1990) noted that 500ml of blood loss does not have a detrimental effect on a woman who is well nourished. This is also the same volume of blood that is taken during blood donation (Burnley *et al* 2006), after which people are offered a cup of tea and a biscuit rather than being considered to have haemorrhaged! Haematologist Gill Gyte (1992) suggested it would be more useful to consider haematological and physical implications of third stage management rather than blood loss alone. She also argues that healthy women appear to cope well with blood losses of up to 1000ml, and suggests that we know very little about the consequences of either very small or heavy blood loss during third stage.

Sara also raised questions about the results of the third stage trials when she noticed that, in contrast to women who experienced physiological placental birth at home, women who had active management in the hospital often lost large blood clots in the toilet on the postnatal ward an hour or two after birth (Wickham 1999). She raised the question of whether the uterotonic drugs were preventing blood loss temporarily and suggested that, if we measured blood loss over a longer period of time, we might see a rather different picture.

As this debate continued, Begley *et al* (2010, 2015) added that, because of blood dilution that occurs during pregnancy, 500ml of blood prior to pregnancy carries the same amount of haemoglobin as around 600-750ml of blood at birth. Anecdotally, a number of researchers and clinicians have pointed out that a woman's blood volume increases by up to 1500ml during pregnancy and that one of the functions of this may be to protect the woman against adverse effects of blood loss during and after the birth.

Nowadays, there is a tendency to separate the definitions of postpartum haemorrhage (blood loss greater than 500ml) from severe post-partum haemorrhage (blood loss greater than 1000ml) and major obstetric haemorrhage (blood loss greater than 1500ml), and this is reflected both in subsequent Cochrane reviews (Begley *et al* 2010, 2015) and the World Health Organization recommendations for the prevention and treatment of postpartum haemorrhage (WHO 2012). However, the WHO (1996) had long noted that even 1000ml is not necessarily excessive in a well-nourished healthy woman and does not need treatment if the woman is well. This idea is now becoming more widely accepted, along with the notion that the definition of postpartum haemorrhage *"…should include both blood loss and clinical signs of cardiovascular changes after delivery."* (Borovac-Pinhiero *et al* 2018).

Another key issue is that, even if there was a consensus on the volume of blood loss that constituted a haemorrhage, research consistently shows that it is incredibly difficult to accurately estimate or measure blood loss (Razvi *et al* 1996, Schorn 2010). This is partly because blood tends to mix with other fluids (such as amniotic fluid) and soak into sheets, pads and other fabrics. We know both from research and from the experience of those who help practitioners develop and test their ability to estimate blood loss in simulations that there is a tendency towards underestimation when blood loss is high, and overestimation when blood loss is low (Razvi *et al* 1996, Bose *et al* 2006, Schorn 2010).

The Bristol third stage trial

One of the first key studies to look at the management of the third stage of labour was carried out in Bristol, England, and the results were published in 1988. A large trial was designed to show whether or not active management of the third stage should be routinely recommended to all women (Prendiville *et al* 1988). The uterotonic used was Syntometrine (5 units Syntocinon plus 0.5 mg ergometrine) given IM, unless women had raised blood pressure, in which case she was given 10 international units of Syntocinon (also IM). The results were published in the British Medical Journal. The authors concluded that active management should continue to be routinely recommended, as blood loss in the women receiving expectant management was significantly higher.

The authors concluded that active management of the third stage reduced the rate of postpartum haemorrhage equal to or greater than 1000ml. The Bristol trial was seen as a landmark study, and the difference in outcomes between the two approaches to the third stage of labour became a key element of the information that midwives and doctors shared with women. Evidence from the Bristol trial is still used as the basis for recommending routine management of the third stage of labour, especially for women with more risk factors or who may be more compromised if they do bleed, for instance because they have a low BMI or haemoglobin level.

However, a number of criticisms of the Bristol trial appeared in both professional and lay journals following the publication of the results. The first of these was that the hospital already had a policy of recommending routine active management of the third stage and, prior to the trial, only six weeks had been allocated for midwives to become familiar and confident in using a physiological approach. At the start of the trial only 13 per cent of the midwives felt very confident in expectant management, and this went up to only 22 per cent after the trial (Begley *et al* 2010). There was debate about whether or not this could have affected the outcomes (Stockdale 1997, Kierse 1998, Featherstone 1999). This is an important question because, in a trial by Begley *et al* (1990), the haemorrhage rate in the expectant management group dropped over the course of the trial from 21 per cent in the pilot study to 12 per cent over the first four months and to 7 per cent in the last six months. This difference was thought to be due to midwives becoming more experienced at facilitating physiological placental birth (Begley *et al* 2015). The rate of haemorrhage may have dropped even further had the midwives continued to gain experience.

Another issue is that women who were already at increased risk of bleeding were included in the Bristol trial. This includes women who had not experienced normal first and second stages of labour, women at known risk of postpartum haemorrhage, women who were given opiate drugs and epidurals and women who had episiotomies. All of these women should have been excluded from the research because this does not give a true result for expectant management in women who had a low risk of excessive bleeding after birth. The argument used at the time was that the researchers did not know for certain if these reasons were justifiable reasons for recommending active management.

A large number of the women (53 per cent) randomised to the expectant management group had neither expectant nor active management. They received a mixed approach including components of active management such as clamping the cord and early cord cutting. For some women, an expectant approach seemed only to mean avoiding the use of Syntometrine (Stevenson 1989, Inch 1990, Gyte 1990, 1991).

It is interesting to note that both the women and midwives involved in the trial preferred active management of the third stage (Harding *et al* 1989). This is not surprising considering that this had been the midwives' usual practice for years, and was a way of working with which they and many women were already comfortable. In addition, because the Bristol trial was a randomised controlled trial (RCT), the group of women who had already stated a preference for physiological birth of the placenta were automatically excluded from the trial, so their views would not have been included. Later research suggested that women are satisfied with whichever form of third stage management they receive (Rogers *et al* 1998). This appears to support the notion that women believe that *'what is must be best'* (Porter & MacIntyre 1984, van Teijlingen *et al* 2003) and many women assume that any care offered must be well thought out (Santalahti *et al* 1998).

There was debate about the methodology and findings of the Bristol trial. Some of the later trials attempted to respond to some of the problems identified in this trial. Thus one of the achievements of the Bristol trial was that it raised many questions and stimulated thinking in this area.

The Dublin and Brighton trials

These trials included women who were considered to be healthy and at low risk of bleeding.

The Dublin trial was carried out by Begley *et al* (1990) in Ireland. Intravenous ergometrine (0.5 mg) was the uterotonic used for woman having a managed third stage, although it is important to note that this is not what was (or is) normally used. Had Syntocinon been used, there may have been fewer adverse effects, as these are known side effects of ergometrine. The results showed that women were statistically less likely to experience excessive bleeding with active management, but had more adverse effects such as increased incidence of raised blood pressure, nausea and vomiting. Interestingly, the results also showed much lower incidences of excessive bleeding in the expectant arm of the trial than in the Bristol study, although it is always difficult to compare data between different trials. There were more retained placentas (and therefore manual removals of placentas) in the group of women who had actively managed third stages of labour.

In the smaller Brighton trial (Thilaganathan *et al* 1993), the main findings were that there was no difference in blood loss between the groups of women having expectant or active management of their third stage. The authors used 1ml of Syntometrine in this trial. Haemoglobin levels were similar in the two groups of women three days after birth. The third stage of labour in this trial was found to be longer in the group of women who had expectant management. The authors of the Cochrane review, however, caution that the findings of this trial might not be reliable due to its size (Begley *et al* 2015).

The Hinchingbrooke trial

Based on their own practice and a desire for more knowledge (see Gyte 1994), researchers carried out the Hinchingbrooke trial (Rogers *et al* 1998). This trial was unusual in that it took place in a hospital where expectant management was more common. However, in questionnaires completed by 92 of the 153 midwives involved in the trial, 84 per cent of them said that they felt 'very confident' in active management, but only 42 per cent of them said that they felt 'very confident' in expectant management (Begley *et al* 2015). The paper on this trial (Rogers *et al* 1998) states that prophylactic oxytocin was given to 19.5 per cent of the women in the intervention group and the other 75 per cent of women in this group received Syntocinon plus ergometrine.

The trial showed that the rate of blood loss over 500ml was two and a half times greater in women who had expectant management (16.5 per cent) compared with women who had active management (6.8 per cent). The findings of the Hinchingbrooke trial were considered more reliable than those of the Bristol trial because some of the women who were at higher risk of having excessive bleeding were not included, and researchers showed that blood loss was still lower with active management even in healthy women.

The difference in blood loss over 1000ml was similar between the two groups though. Severe (over 1000ml) bleeding occurred in 2.6 per cent of the women who had expectant management and in 1.7 per cent of the women who had active management; a difference that isn't statistically significant. There was no difference in the number of retained placentas. Women who had expectant management had slightly heavier babies, and it was thought that this was because their babies received their full quota of blood while the cord was still pulsating after birth (Rogers *et al* 1998, Rogers & Wood 1999). At the time of this research however, 'delayed' cord clamping was not the norm for women having active management of the third stage of labour.

Debating the issues

Once these first few trials had been published, it was generally accepted that active management of the third stage was preferable and should be recommended for all women. Over the next few years, most of the subsequent studies and trials focused on which drugs should be used and the relative merits of the different elements of active management (for instance Khan *et al* 1997, Ramirez *et al* 2001, Vasegh *et al* 2005, Hoffman *et al* 2006, Jerbi *et al* 2007, Gülmezoglu *et al* 2009, Kashanian *et al* 2010). Given that this places the focus firmly on how active management should be conducted (rather than whether it should be conducted), their findings may not be helpful for women and practitioners who want to know about the relative harms and benefits of the three different approaches to the birth of the placenta.

At the same time, however, a number of debates were going on in the midwifery and medical literature, and many other interesting conversations were happening. The ideas which underpin some of these will be considered further in chapter 6, when we talk about the wider issues. First, we will consider the conclusions reached by the authors of the main and most recent systematic review in this area, when they put together the randomised controlled trials that had been carried out.

The Cochrane review

There have been a number of systematic reviews of this area, of which the most useful, comprehensive and respected are published by the Cochrane Collaboration. The most recent Cochrane review of active versus expectant management for women in the third stage of labour was written by Begley *et al* (2015). The review authors found eight studies suitable for inclusion, and these studies involved a total of 8,892 women.

All but one of these studies were carried out in high-income countries; four of the studies compared active with expectant management while the other four compared active versus a mixture of managements.

Probably the most important thing to know at the outset is that the evidence is not considered to be of high quality. As we have noted in earlier sections of our book, there were some methodological problems in some of the studies, and this needs to be taken into account when considering the findings.

In simple terms, the authors found that, *"…for all women, irrespective of their risk of severe bleeding, active management reduced severe bleeding and anaemia. However, it also reduced the baby's birthweight and increased the mother's blood pressure, after-pains, vomiting and the number of women returning to hospital with bleeding."* (Begley *et al* 2015). So there are risks and benefits with active, expectant and physiological approaches to the third stage and with different uterotonic drugs. Women who have one or more of the risk factors that we described in chapter 4 may wish to weigh these up particularly carefully in relation to their individual circumstances.

The findings are slightly different for low risk (or healthy) women. *"For women at low risk of bleeding, findings were similar though there was no difference in risk of severe bleeding."* (Begley *et al* 2015). In other words, there is no real benefit to active management in terms of severe bleeding (by which we mean blood loss greater than 1000ml) for 'low risk' women. There does appear to be a benefit for healthy women in that active management reduces the chance of bleeding more than 500ml and less than 1000ml. The Cochrane authors offer further information in this regard:

"In high-income countries with high levels of clinician expertise and adequate access to emergency care, healthy women do not appear to suffer unduly from the results of above average blood loss (about 500mL) that does not reach the level of severe primary postpartum haemorrhage (PPH) (greater than 1000ml) (Bloomfield 1990). For example, this

review found only a small number of low-risk women (29 out of 3134, 0.9%) had a sufficiently large blood loss to require a blood transfusion." (Begley *et al* 2015).

One important consideration is that blood transfusions are not given unless really warranted nowadays, and it can't be assumed that the absence of a blood transfusion means that the woman is in good health. A woman may experience other less quantifiable consequences such as tiredness/lethargy or problems establishing breast feeding. These women may be prescribed iron tablets which can cause digestive problems such as constipation, which can be particularly uncomfortable for women who have perineal bruising, tears and/or sutures.

Another consideration, as the authors have noted in several reviews (Begley *et al* 2010, 2015), is that all of these trials took place in hospitals where active management was the norm and, as we have noted elsewhere, if practitioners are knowledgeable and skilled in active management but less so in expectant management, this may make a difference to the outcomes in the studies. It is also interesting to note that, in one study, the mean blood loss among the group of women who had active management was more than in the group of women who had expectant management in another study.

From a research perspective, and because our knowledge has changed over the past few years (since several of the included studies were carried out), the authors point out that, *"Given the concerns about early cord clamping and the potential adverse effects of some uterotonics, it is critical now to look at the individual components of third stage management."* (Begley *et al* 2015). Ultimately, the authors of this Cochrane review share our view that, *"Women should be given information on the benefits and harms of both methods to support informed choice."* (Begley *et al* 2015).

6. Wider issues

In the previous chapter, we discussed the research trials that have been carried out on third stage management as well as the most recent systematic review which has examined these trials. One significant and ongoing issue relates to the limitations of these research studies. Key concerns include the way that expectant management was defined in these trials, the environment within which birth took place and the practices which were associated with it. These practices, as we noted early in chapter 5, may be different from the way that a midwife would facilitate physiological birth of the placenta in a setting and situation conducive to physiological birth.

This chapter discusses a number of wider issues relating to the birth of the placenta, including uncertainties, questions that need to be researched, related practices, decision making and other thinking on this subject.

Other approaches to research

Midwives and others have long questioned the way in which care during the third stage of labour has been researched. For instance, around the same time that the Bristol trial was being conducted, midwife Barbara Watson carried out a very small, retrospective research project involving 100 women at a hospital in England (Watson 1990). Half of the women experienced expectant management and half had active management. She found that haemoglobin levels after three days were similar among all the women in the trial and concluded that expectant management is appropriate for some women (Watson 1990). At the time of the research this hospital already had an expectant management rate of 17 per cent, so the midwives were already competent and confident with this approach.

Watson's study used haemoglobin levels rather than blood loss as an outcome measure. As we suggested before, it may be more helpful to consider women's holistic wellbeing rather than just focusing on blood loss alone. Wellbeing can to some extent be measured through haemoglobin levels, although we could also consider factors such as shortness of breath, heart rate, blood pressure, tiredness, dizziness, fainting and the woman's ability to care for her baby, including breast feeding.

Two really interesting studies were published in 2012. These were not randomised controlled trials, but this is not a bad thing, as different types of research can show us different things. The first was carried out in England by Nove *et al* (2012). These researchers compared the rates of postpartum haemorrhage in more than half a million healthy women who gave birth at home and in hospital. They found that more women who intended to give birth in hospital had a blood loss of more than 1000ml compared to women who intended to give birth at home. This may be because the type of birth was also different; blood loss is likely to be associated with more obstetric drugs and interventions, such as induction of labour, augmentation (speeding up labour with a drip), episiotomy, instrumental delivery and caesarean section.

Davis *et al* (2012) carried out a study in New Zealand and found that more women lost more than 1000ml with active management (as compared to physiological placental birth) no matter where they gave birth. So these results are a little different from those of Nove *et al* (2012) and we can't determine from either of the studies exactly why a homelike environment and physiological placental birth seem to lead to better outcomes in healthy women. But the results support the idea (which we have mentioned a few times) that environment, ideology and the type of care that a woman receives can make a significant difference.

As we have shown throughout the book, the issues relating to the evidence are complex. It is also the case that people interpret evidence differently. There are certainly many people who believe that the evidence supports a routine recommendation of active management of the third stage of labour, but others do not agree. We have looked at the difference between women who are healthy and have had a straightforward labour and birth and women who have risk factors or who have experienced intervention during their labour or the birth of their baby. Active management of the third stage of labour is more necessary in hospitals because women are more likely to experience excessive bleeding because of the higher rates of intervention in hospitals.

We need more research into out-of-hospital settings, including research embodying midwifery knowledge and skills and valuing physiology. It would be immensely helpful to continue to study physiological placental birth among women who give birth at home or in home-like settings with midwives skilled at facilitating undisturbed birth and physiological placental birth.

Midwives who are experienced in supporting women to have physiological placental births emphasise the value of trusting relationships. Getting to know women enables midwives to discuss birth, build the woman's confidence and suggest any appropriate dietary and/or lifestyle changes that might help her stay healthy, grow a healthy baby and placenta and have as straightforward a birth as possible. It enables midwives to understand in more detail whether the woman is more likely to bleed after birth and consider what steps she could take during pregnancy that might reduce the chances of this happening. This may be through diet or lifestyle changes, or by building trust and providing an unhurried, relaxing environment for her to birth in. Trust and mutual understanding through continuity of carer enables the woman and midwife to work together during labour and birth to increase the likelihood of birth unfolding without complication. Importantly, in the unlikely event of a problem, or a bleed during or after the birth of the placenta, this trust enables them to work together easily and efficiently to deal with any emergency safely and as quickly as possible.

Different ways of knowing

A difficulty that arises when we base practice purely on the results of randomised controlled trials is that these can disregard crucial elements of knowledge. Well designed and expertly carried out research trials can give us good information about treatments and practices involving large groups of people. However, they tell us little about individuals, about the differences between people and about the subtle effects of treatments and procedures.

Kathleen Fahy (2009) also questioned whether or not a randomised controlled trial could be done on third stage management, because women should only be randomised after the birth of the baby. It is only at this point that it is clear whether or not a woman has had a physiological labour and birth and is at lower risk of bleeding. Fahy suggests that it would be unethical to randomise women at this stage of labour. Other researchers believe that randomisation should happen as close to the intervention as possible, and that this could occur just before the birth of the baby, as long as the woman has had full information during pregnancy and gives her consent again during labour. These researchers acknowledge the ethical difficulties of informed consent but argue that, without trial evidence, clinicians will do what they believe to be best. Some experienced midwives and others studying physiology have expressed concern that asking women to think about different third stage approaches and give consent during this crucial phase of labour might in itself be an intervention that impacts on delicate hormonal changes and thus the birth process.

There is increasing interest in the hormonal flow of birth (Uvnäs Moberg 2011, Buckley 2015) and in the consequences of giving synthetic oxytocin to birthing women. Sarah Buckley (2015) has brought together a body of research on this topic and highlights concerns about the routine use of synthetic oxytocin.

We are also beginning to see the emergence of further

studies which, while not on the topic of the third stage of labour, add knowledge which may be relevant to women who are making decisions about this. For instance, Grotegut *et al* (2011) looked at women who had experienced excessive bleeding which was related to their uterus not contracting well after the birth. The researchers compared the amounts of synthetic oxytocin that had been given to women during labour who had excessive bleeding after birth, and the amount given to women who had not experienced excessive bleeding after birth, but who were similar in other ways. The results showed that the women who had excessive bleeding had been given more than two and a half times the amount of synthetic oxytocin during labour than the other women. The researchers carried out a number of statistical tests which indicated that this was not due to other differences such as induction of labour, body mass index (BMI) or race. In other words, when women are given substantial amounts of oxytocin during labour, this has a detrimental effect on the ability of their uterine muscle to effectively contract after birth. As Buckley (2015) found in her analysis of the research on oxytocin, being given synthetic oxytocin during one birth may negatively affect a woman's subsequent births as well. As we have previously mentioned, Buckley's (2011, 2015) work also highlights how physiological birth of the placenta could benefit women and their babies in terms of the immediate and ongoing interaction between them through bonding, breast feeding and wellbeing.

Research is only one way of knowing, and it has long been understood that this is simply one element of evidence-based practice (Sackett 1996). Experience and observation are often a catalyst for research, as they lead us to raise questions about things that we notice. But they are also crucial in practice, as the limitations of research leave large gaps which need to be filled by those making decisions and those attending them.

For example, one midwife described an unusual incident of a woman having a velamentous insertion of the cord (where the vessels of the cord separate and go through the membranes before reaching the placenta). The midwife knew the woman, had been with her during two previous births, knew that the pattern of her labour was unusual for her and encouraged her to follow her instincts despite the unusually slow, stop-start progress of her labour. The midwife was reminded of Australian GP John Stevenson's observation that this can be a sign of the body taking care of a problem with the cord – such as a knot. The midwife refrained from intervening with the normal course of labour and the baby was born healthy and well. Only after the arrival of the placenta was the midwife able to understand the problem. It is possible that any of the standard medical interventions for a 'prolonged' labour could have seriously compromised the baby and may even have been fatal (Wolford 1997). While we need to be cautious of anecdotal experiences and mindful not to think that single occurrences are representative of a wider trend, the history of science shows us that many of our most useful discoveries emerged from a single idea or intuition that later became the subject of deeper investigation.

We still have some way to go in balancing different forms of knowledge, and have much to learn from midwives and doctors who have incorporated openness to different ways of knowing in their own practice and who listen to women, observe carefully, and treat each woman as an individual. We will return to this in the final section of this chapter, but before we do that we would like to explore some of the issues raised earlier in more depth.

Returning to the question of normal blood loss

Some midwives believe that by considering the theory and their experience of physiology, we could gain a better understanding of issues which currently lack good research evidence. As we mentioned in chapter 5, one of us (Sara) described her observations when she briefly worked on a hospital postnatal ward after having been a home birth midwife experienced in physiological placental birth. She noticed that the women who had had actively managed third stages often lost large blood clots when they first visited the toilet 2-3 hours after having given birth.

"I realised that their blood loss was probably more noticeable to me because I had previously been practising in a situation in which the majority of women chose physiological third stage. After a physiological third stage, the women did not have the pattern of heavy bleeding delayed for a few hours after the birth that I was observing in the women who had had active management in the hospital. It struck me that this might account for the different amounts of blood lost between women who had physiological and managed third stage. Could the use of an oxytocic inhibit the normal blood loss at birth, but cause the blood to be somehow retained by the woman's body and expelled later? This would account both for the difference in recorded blood loss at birth and the later loss of blood in women experiencing active management. Physiologically, this would make sense. The use of an oxytocic drug causes a strong and sustained contraction of the uterus. The uterus is too well contracted to release a large amount of blood at this stage, which is why the blood loss is smaller in most cases." (Wickham 1999: 14)

The article quoted above also questioned whether or not it is preferable to minimise blood loss, given that it may be normal physiology for some women to lose more blood than others. And because a woman's blood volume increases during pregnancy, blood loss after birth is part of the return to normal physiology:

"...if the woman's body is physiologically adapted to losing more blood, it wouldn't be until the effects of the oxytocic had started to wear off that the uterus would be able to relax sufficiently to achieve this. So it may be that the average amount of blood lost during physiological third stage is "normal", while the lesser amounts of blood lost during active management are abnormally low. If we recorded the

amount of lochia [blood] *lost in the first few hours after birth together with that lost during the birth itself, would the figures for the two types of third stage correlate more closely? Could it be that the total blood loss in women experiencing active management might actually be higher?"* (Wickham 1999: 15)

As above, the hypothesis that active management may lead to more blood loss than is counted in the research trials is supported by the findings of Begley *et al* (2015) who cite the increased likelihood of women who have experienced active management returning to the hospital in the postnatal period because of excessive bleeding. However, this may be because other medical interventions have led to a greater likelihood of infection or secondary postpartum haemorrhage.

The impact of environment and ideology

We have already mentioned that all of the research trials making comparisons between different ways of managing the third stage of labour have been carried out in hospitals with practices based on obstetric ideology and that some people believe that the environment of care (which includes who is with a woman at birth) may be an important factor in the outcome of the birth of the placenta.

One of the first studies through which we can explore this was carried out in New Zealand. In a small, exploratory study, Prichard *et al* (1995) looked at 213 women who had home births. The emphasis was on the lack of disturbance to the physiological processes of birth, and the results showed that only 3.3 per cent of the women had a postpartum haemorrhage (which in this study was defined as a blood loss over 500ml). None of the women required a manual removal of their placenta. No woman had a reported blood loss of more than 900ml. However, the researchers acknowledged that estimated blood loss can be inaccurate and that the methods used in this research may have introduced bias.

They concluded that it raised important issues for exploration rather than providing definitive answers.

One of the difficulties with research into the third stage of labour is that it can be difficult to separate out the impact of the birth attendant, the setting and the beliefs of all of those involved. So it is useful to have research like that carried out by Logue (1990), who looked specifically at the impact of the individual practitioner on the occurrence of postpartum haemorrhage. In this study, it was discovered that, in one particular hospital, the postpartum haemorrhage rate varied from 1-16 per cent for midwives and 1-31 per cent for registrars (obstetric doctors in training). Women cared for by doctors and midwives who were considered to be 'heavy-handed' were more likely to have a postpartum haemorrhage. This was also seen during the Hinchingbrooke third stage trial, as Rogers and Wood (2003) discussed.

The Cochrane reviewers (Begley *et al* 2015) suggest that the skill of the practitioner is a crucial factor in supporting physiological birth of the placenta. The review cites observational studies in The Netherlands (Bais *et al* 2004) and New Zealand (NZCOM 2009) where midwives may be more skilled in physiological placental birth than in some other areas. These studies showed that there was no reduction in blood loss among the women who had their third stages actively managed. In the New Zealand study, 33,752 women were included. All had physiological labours and births. Almost half of these women had physiological third stages and their blood loss was slightly less than the women who had active management of the third stage of labour (Begley *et al* 2015).

A useful addition to the literature on placental birth comes from Australia (Fahy *et al* 2010). This retrospective cohort study (which looks at what happened to a group of women depending on whether they had one or other type of third stage) included 3436 women who were at low risk of postpartum haemorrhage, who had no interventions during labour and birth and no predisposing factors for excessive bleeding after birth. Of these women, 3075 gave birth in a tertiary unit (a large obstetric unit) and 361 of these women gave birth in a free standing midwifery unit. The researchers compared 'holistic psychophysiological care' with active management of the third stage of labour. The 'holistic psychophysiological care' was described in contrast to the usual 'expectant care', and included creating a conducive environment in which the woman feels: *"…safe, secure, cared about and trusting that her privacy is respected. The attending midwife must be knowledgeable and feel confident about optimising psychophysiology during the third stage of labour."* (Fahy *et al* 2010: 147-148).

This includes; *"…immediate and sustained skin-to-skin contact between the woman and the baby who are both kept warm; the midwife gently encourages the woman to focus on her baby whilst maintaining awareness that the placenta is yet to be born; the support people remain focused on mother and baby; there is 'self-attachment' breastfeeding; the midwife unobtrusively observes for signs of separation of the placenta; there is no fundal massage or meddling; the placenta is birthed entirely by maternal effort and gravity. The midwife or the woman gently 'checks the fundus' for 1h* [one hour] *post placental birth to ensure contraction and haemostasis* [stopping of bleeding]*."* (Fahy *et al* 2010: 148).

Most of the 3075 women who were at low risk of bleeding too much after birth and who gave birth in the tertiary unit received active management, and 344 women had blood losses over 500ml (11.2 per cent). Most of the 361 women who had their babies in the free standing midwifery led unit had 'psychophysiological' care and ten of them had blood losses of over 500ml (2.8 per cent). So in this study, women who birthed in the midwifery unit were less likely to lose more than 500ml of blood than similar women who birthed in the tertiary unit.

The researchers also compared the type of third stage, no matter where the woman gave birth. This showed that, of the 3016 women who had active management, 347 had blood losses of over 500ml (11.5 per cent) and of the 420 women who received psychophysiological care seven had blood losses of over 500ml (1.7 per cent). So the women who had psychophysiological care were less likely to bleed heavily than the women who had active management even if they were in the tertiary unit. The number of women who had blood losses of over 1000ml, or of over 1500ml was extremely small, but was slightly higher in women who had active management in the tertiary unit.

The researchers concluded that holistic psychophysiological care for the third stage of labour is safe for women who are at low risk of bleeding excessively after birth. While the researchers acknowledge that there are limitations to their study and suggest more research needs to be done, this would seem to confirm the importance of the ideology and environment of care.

Placental birth in water

As our understanding of the benefits of water during labour and/or birth grows, more women are deciding to labour in water and some remain in water for the birth. We have observed that there is some variation in the practices around the birth of women's placentas where they have given birth in water. In many maternity units and in some community settings, women are asked to leave the pool for the birth of their placenta. There are various reasons why women are asked to do this. Some practitioners are concerned about not being able to measure blood loss. However, midwife colleagues suggest that it is possible to have a reasonable sense of this from the colour of the water.

Another concern is that it might be difficult to get a woman out of the pool quickly enough in the case of a sudden postpartum haemorrhage but, again, other practitioners point out that this is a relatively rare event and that there may be advantages to remaining in the pool which need to be balanced against possible disadvantages. The level of concern depends on the midwife's knowledge, skill and confidence, and these concerns may be exacerbated when women and midwives do not know each other before labour.

Other reasons given for asking women to leave the pool may be a consequence of the myth that waterbirth is associated with a hypothetical risk of water embolism (see Wickham 2005) and/or because midwives are not easily able to administer an oxytocic and/or perform the manoeuvres associated with active management while women remain in the pool. However, we can find no evidence to suggest that it is better for women to leave the pool for the birth of the placenta rather than stay in it.

Some midwives have a concern about keeping the baby warm enough if the woman stays in the pool to birth the placenta. Many midwives encourage the woman to keep the baby's body submerged, but this is easier to facilitate in some situations than others. Another concern shared by some practitioners is that staying in the pool for the birth of the placenta can lead to a delay in assessing whether the woman has had a tear and whether she might benefit from suturing.

The usual practice of midwives who are experienced at facilitating physiological placental birth is to follow the woman's lead as far as staying in or getting out of the pool is concerned, unless she appears to be bleeding more than usual. The midwife is then likely to ask her to get out of the pool in order to better assess the blood loss and discuss possible treatment. Unless there is a problem, any interruption at this delicate time may disrupt the birth of the placenta, and should be avoided unless necessary.

Placenta rituals

There is a wide range of variation in how different parents feel about seeing, touching or doing something significant or symbolic with their placenta after the birth. Some people like to look at it and learn about how it worked to sustain their baby, or perhaps to marvel at its structure. Some parents want the midwife to take it away immediately. Others want to keep the placenta. Some have plans and know what they want to do with it, while some parents take it home, pop it in the freezer and leave it there for a while (sometimes years!) before they decide. There are now books available which explore these issues and offer really interesting perspectives on the meaning of the placenta (Lim 2015, Jordan 2017). In this section, we will briefly share a few examples of placenta rituals for those who are interested in this. Some parents carry out more than one ritual (for instance, taking a placenta print and then burying the placenta and planting a tree) but some of these rituals involve destroying or consuming the placenta, so parents need to pick one or the other. As with everything, if you like the idea of one or more of these rituals then we would encourage you to find out as much as possible beforehand so that you are prepared and fully informed before you begin.

The first set of rituals could be described as **placenta art**, as they involve creating some sort of creative project with the placenta. One example is placenta printing, where paint (or, occasionally, the blood that remains on the placenta after birth) is put over the placenta. The placenta is then pressed onto paper, fabric, canvas or another medium to create a lasting print. This may then be framed or made into something else.

Another option is **placenta burial**, where the placenta is placed into the ground, sometimes as part of a ceremony, sometimes with a simple thank you for sustaining the baby's life and sometimes with a tree (often a fruit tree) or other symbolic plant placed over the burial area. In some families, this then becomes the baby's tree. Such rituals do not have to be carried out immediately after birth, as the placenta can be frozen for a long time in a suitable container. Indeed, we know of families who have frozen their babies' placentas for months or years because they wanted to wait until they moved into the house that would be their long-term home.

A further option is **placenta consumption** (also known as placentophagy) where a woman eats her placenta. Placentas are consumed in a number of forms; raw (either as chunks or blended into a smoothie), fried up (sometimes with onions), cooked into a meal (we know of stew, lasagne and pâté recipes) or dehydrated, chopped and encapsulated. The latter is becoming an increasingly popular option amongst some women, and there is a range of views about the value of this (Wickham 2015).

Proponents of placenta consumption claim that the consumption of placenta promotes postnatal recovery, but most of the information on this is anecdotal and based on personal experience. It could be that the placebo effect is in play here and, while this is not necessarily a bad thing (in that anything that helps women to feel good after birth should be welcomed and celebrated), we need to be mindful of giving accurate, evidence-based information to woman and families.

Detractors claim that placental consumption carries risks, which include the transmission of infection and interference with breast milk production (Farr *et al* 2016). Currently, there is not much basis to most of these claims either, and we need more research into this area (Coyle *et al* 2015). Those who are speaking out against placentophagy tend to cite a single case or example (where there may be many other factors that could have affected a particular outcome) or a general concern which isn't backed up by the findings of research.

A recent review of the experiences of over 23,000 women who ate their placentas or placenta products did not show any adverse outcomes (Benyshek *et al* 2018). However, as this research analysed existing medical records rather than collecting and comparing prospective data, it would be useful to have more research into this topic. The debate (and divide) on placentophagy is likely to continue for some time and this is an area which a lot of people are currently writing about. As we write, the conversation seems to be becoming more polarised and, as with many areas, we suspect that the truth is probably somewhere in the middle of the extremes.

Lotus birth

Lotus birth *"…is the practice of leaving the umbilical cord uncut, so that the baby remains attached to his or her placenta until the cord naturally separates at the umbilicus, exactly as a cut cord does, at three to ten days after birth."* (Buckley 2005: 40). Women who have experienced lotus birth often report that the cord separates more quickly following lotus birth than when the cord is clamped and cut and a small stump is left to fall off after a few days.

While there appear to be no early written records about the practice of lotus birth, it is practised among some aboriginal peoples. It has also been documented in observations of chimpanzees, but the first written account among humans may be in 1974, when Clair Lotus Day from California decided to leave her baby's cord attached to her baby and placenta until it separated by itself (Buckley 2005, Zinsser 2017).

Lotus birth is promoted by some mothers, birth activists, educators and midwives as a *"…logical extension of natural childbirth* [which] *invites us to reclaim the so-called third stage of labour for our babies and ourselves, and to honour the placenta, our babies' first source of nourishment."* (Buckley 2005: 41).

Benefits are believed to include a slower and gentler transition for the baby into life outside its mother's womb, a time of rest and seclusion for the mother and her baby and immediate family (Lim 2015, Zinsser 2017). This is because, if the baby and placenta remain attached, the mother is more likely to stay at home. Many of the women who choose lotus birth like the fact that the baby is less likely to be 'passed around'. This is partly because it is more difficult to handle the baby and the placenta, and partly because some people do not like the idea of the placenta still being attached. Either way, the mother gets to spend more time with her baby. Lotus birth is also considered an acknowledgement of the spiritual aspects of birth and the placenta (Lim 2015). Finally, proponents suggest that there may be a reduction in infection of the cord (Buckley 2005). Michel Odent has noted that lotus birth "*usefully reverses the cultural conditioning that cutting the cord is physiologically necessary.*" (Davis 2010: 177).

Lotus birth is more often practised at home births, but there is no reason why women should not keep baby, cord and placenta intact and together wherever they give birth and lotus birth has been known to occur after a planned caesarean birth (Davies 2007).

A number of anecdotal accounts recommend different ways of looking after the cord and placenta during the time they remain attached to the baby. Some suggest wiping or washing the placenta after birth, then liberally salting the placenta and adding drops of lavender or some other antiseptic, pleasant herbal preparation. Some suggest keeping the placenta dry and in a bowl or sieve and exposed to air without adding salt, while others suggest putting the placenta in a cloth bag (sometimes with salt) and wrapping baby and placenta in a shawl. The placenta has been described as developing a musky smell by some, but others do not experience this. The cord, like the placenta, gradually dries and shrivels, and the cord usually hardens and then separates. It is worth noting, however, that this process may occur differently depending on the climate. Many of these accounts also provide tips on how to handle the baby while still attached to its cord and placenta (Buckley 2005, Zenack 1998, Lim 2015, Zinsser 2017).

Cord tying, banding or burning

Another area in which it would be fascinating to go back in time and see what our foremothers did relates to the question of how one ties off or otherwise restricts the umbilical cord after it has been cut in order to prevent the baby from losing blood. In reality, the cord only needs to be secured in this way for a few hours, but in modern systems of maternity care the plastic clamp is often left on until the cord falls off after a few days. But a small number of parents and care providers have begun to explore (or perhaps, more accurately, revisit) other ways of restricting the blood in the cord.

The main issue that some people have with the modern plastic cord clamps is that they are hard and may be uncomfortable for the baby, especially if they get accidentally caught and pull the cord. A smaller but equally important issue for some parents is that these clamps are deemed clinical, impersonal and not very environmentally friendly in comparison to some of the alternatives.

One option that is used by some midwives involves using a device which looks a bit like eyelash curlers to put a band (usually made of latex, which is 'greener' than plastic but a common source of allergy) over the cord. The band sits tightly around the cord, restricting blood loss, and as nothing protrudes from the cord, it cannot be accidentally jarred or pulled. It can be snipped off with a pair of scissors but is quite tight so, as long as the band is applied correctly, it isn't very likely to fall off by accident.

Another alternative is to put a tie around the cord. This method is likely to have been used in many traditional societies and is still in use or being revived in some cultures. One example of this is a muka or flax fibre cord tie, traditionally used by Aotearoa Maori people in New Zealand. Muka is environmentally friendly, considered to have antibacterial properties and is softer than a plastic cord clamp. But some midwives and mothers make cord ties out of woven wool or thread and a variety of natural or other materials are used. Some people take the time to pick colours and invest something of themselves into the crafting of this item for a baby. While such fibres may not contain the antibacterial properties of muka, the tie can be boiled before use to ensure that it is clean (although birth itself is not sterile).

Care must be taken with the knots that are used with any form of cord tying. The cord should neither be tied too tightly (because this can cause a tear in the cord) or too loosely (as a poorly tied knot and/or the existence of loose ends can lead to the tie being pulled off and allow bleeding to occur). Because there is a small risk of tearing the cord, ties are usually made from a few strands of thread (such as embroidery thread) woven or plaited together. Using something slightly thicker means that the tie will be less likely to tear the cord when it is tightened and knotted.

The final possibility (although we are sure that more will emerge or come to our attention by the time we next update this book) is to burn the cord. If a cord is burned, then no tie or clamp is needed, as the process effectively cauterises or seals the blood vessels. A box is usually used, and the cord is laid across it so that candles can be used to burn through the cord. A box or plate can be used to keep the flame away from the mother and baby, and catch the drips of wax which will fall from the candles, especially if tapered candles are used. This is not a fast process; the cord can take up to fifteen minutes to burn through. Cord burning is generally used by people opting for home birth, as hospitals won't allow naked flames, but proponents of this describe it as a lovely ritual which can involve the whole family.

Regardless of which of these you prefer, it is certainly interesting to consider the vast difference between the two seconds taken to snip the cord when a plastic clamp is applied and the much longer process of burning through a cord. If you are considering an alternative method of severing (or, indeed, not severing) the cord, we would encourage you to find out as much as possible and ensure that you have everything that you will need to hand before you begin. As with many areas of maternity care, you will encounter some extreme views. On the one hand, there are paediatricians who tell horror stories about babies who bled after a cord tie fell off, but there are also people who promote cord tying or burning without acknowledging that there are things you need to know and take into account in order to do these safely and in a manner that will be relaxing and joyful for all concerned.

Women and decision making

No matter what the research evidence or any practitioner, policy, guideline or protocol says about the birth of the placenta, it is up to the woman to make the decisions about all and any of her maternity care (Beech 2014, Wickham 2018b). It is also important to remember that caregivers cannot give drugs or perform manoeuvres without the consent of the woman, and some women choose to wait longer, as long as they are not experiencing bleeding or other problems. In this section, we will look at a few of the things that women may want to consider when they weigh up the options and discuss some of the elements of informed decision making.

Over the past few decades, as birth has come to be seen in some settings as a medical event, women have often known little about the birth of the placenta (Green *et al* 1998, Begley *et al* 2015), but Begley *et al* (2015) noted that women are now asking their midwives more questions about the birth of their placenta. Women should be able to talk about the birth of the placenta with a midwife and receive as much information as they want during pregnancy. This should include detailed information about both the benefits and harms of different approaches to placental birth. Women who are considering expectant management or physiological birth of the placenta should also know that the components of active management can be used as treatment if it becomes necessary. Women who are more likely to bleed too much after birth, or who prefer active management should be aware of the potential benefits of delayed cord clamping for their babies.

Women should not be expected to consider the pros and cons of third stage approaches for the first time during labour or after the baby's birth. Neither should women be asked to tick a box during pregnancy expressing their preference without having been given information upon which to base this decision. There should also be a clear and good reason for any intervention that is suggested, as no intervention is without risk. Good communication between the mother and her attendant is important for good decision making and therefore for the mother and the baby's well-being.

There are a number of wider issues which women might want to consider when making their decision. One important factor arising from the research that we have discussed is that there is significant variation in midwives' and doctors' ideology and practice around birth. Individual practitioners might be more aligned with holistic care that supports undisturbed birth where possible, or may be more aligned to an obstetric approach that is more likely to manage the birth process. These ideologies and practices will usually extend to the birth of the woman's placenta.

Because maternity care systems are currently dominated by obstetric ideology, some health care practitioners lack the knowledge, skill and experience needed to help women birth their placentas physiologically (Begley 2014). In research from the UK, Diane Farrar and her colleagues (2010) found that 93 per cent of doctors and 73 per cent of midwives *"always or usually"* advise active management of the third stage of labour. Selfe and Walsh (2015) found evidence that healthy women were not being offered a truly informed choice when it came to the third stage of labour. The women in this study reported that the information they received favoured active management. This is in conflict with the recommendations of a number of bodies. For instance, although NICE in the UK still recommends advising women to have active management, it also explicitly acknowledges that women who are at low risk of excessive bleeding should be supported to have physiological management if they wish (NICE 2017a). The Cochrane review suggests that women should be informed about the benefits and harms of active management and that their decisions should be supported (Begley *et al* 2015).

As we discussed in chapter 4, there are conditions and circumstances that might increase the likelihood of bleeding after birth. These are often listed in midwifery books, obstetric guidelines, in research papers and elsewhere. Sometimes these lists are extensive but, as we noted earlier, we don't always have enough evidence about whether and how these conditions are linked with a higher chance of bleeding. Such lists include women who have had synthetic oxytocic drugs during labour, women who have a blood clotting disorder, fibroids or an unusually-shaped uterus, who experienced antepartum haemorrhage (bleeding during pregnancy), who have anaemia, who are expecting more than one baby (a multiple birth), or who had a long (prolonged) labour or a very fast (precipitate) labour. This list also includes women who have had postpartum haemorrhage or another third stage problem such as retained placenta in a previous labour and birth, but it is important to bear in mind that such problems may have been caused by inappropriate intervention and women may wish to discuss their experiences with a midwife or doctor.

It is impossible to make definitive statements about such things, in part because women are individuals and the conditions we mention above may be more or less serious depending on the woman and circumstances. In most of these situations, many practitioners automatically recommend active management, but women have the right to make their own decisions (Beech 2014). It is often helpful for a woman in a complex situation and who wishes to avoid the use of oxytocic drugs and/or other interventions to discuss this fully with a midwife who is knowledgeable and confident.

It appears that more women would choose a

physiological or expectant approach if they were offered more information and choice. At Hinchingbrooke Hospital, where one of the third stage trials was carried out, researchers commented that, where expectant management is offered as a genuine option, many women will choose it (Rogers *et al* 1998, Rogers & Wood 1999). Our experience is that this is still true today and that many women say they would like the option.

Towards a more holistic approach

As we have mentioned throughout this book, much of the research we have so far tells us only about what happens during third stage when women are in hospitals and receiving fragmented care from practitioners who they have not met before. Many women experience other medical interventions before birthing their placentas.

Many of the issues that we have addressed in this book are symptomatic of larger problems which some people have identified within our culture in general and in modern maternity care in particular (Kirkham 2018a, 2018b). One example is the question of how we define normality, and who we decide is 'normal' and 'not normal'. There are also important questions to be asked about how birth is 'managed', how maternity services are organised, where women are able to give birth, who controls and makes decisions about those things and how all of this relates to women's own agency and their right to make decisions about their bodies, births and experiences (Murphy-Lawless 1998, Edwards *et al* 2018).

Midwives who are experienced in both practice and research have been developing and articulating a midwifery approach to birth which understands the importance of the woman's and baby's health and the impact of environmental, emotional, psychological and social as well as physical factors (Fahy 2009, Hastie 2011). Crucially, practitioners who follow such an approach respect the fact that the physiology of birth is intricate, delicate and woven together throughout the woman's birthing journey. The birth of the placenta doesn't occur in isolation, but within the context of a woman's life journey, at the end of her pregnancy, following her labour and the birth of her baby. In particular, any interference and disturbance during labour and birth can impact on whether or not the woman is able to give birth to her placenta physiologically (Buckley 2015).

The research in this area so far comes from the Netherlands (Bais *et al* 2004), New Zealand (NZCOM 2009) and Australia (Fahy *et al* 2010). We mentioned these earlier in chapter 5. The New Zealand study was a large retrospective study of nearly 34,000 women, many of whom who gave birth with known midwives. This research showed no increase in bleeding when the woman gave birth to her placenta physiologically. However, we know that it may not provide accurate findings as it used medical records to gather the data. The Australian study was a cohort study of nearly 3,500 women who gave birth in a birth centre or in an obstetric unit. Again, this was not a prospective trial, but the number of women included was large and the results were similar. These studies showed that healthy women who were looked after by midwives with a holistic approach, in environments conducive to women being able to respond to their bodies and maintain their hormonal flow gave birth safely to their placentas themselves without the help of oxytocic drugs or other components of active management. The Australian research in particular suggested that women might lose less blood when looked after holistically and enabled to birth their placentas themselves.

We don't yet know enough about how relational care impacts on physiological placental birth, especially when women give birth at home or in midwifery run, freestanding birth centres. We do know that relational care from midwives that encourages women and midwives to build trusting relationships has many positive impacts for mothers and babies (Sandall *et al* 2016). Research from the Albany Midwifery Practice in London, England showed a relatively high rate of physiological placental births and a low rate of postpartum haemorrhage among women with and without medical, obstetric and social challenges (Homer *et al* 2017). Most women in this practice were looked after throughout pregnancy, labour, birth and beyond by a midwife they knew and trusted and nearly 50 per cent gave birth at home.

It is reassuring that it was so clear in Cecily Begley's (1990) research that midwives became increasingly skilled at supporting women to have expectant management of the third stage of labour as they gained experience in this. You might remember from chapter 5 that fewer and fewer women had excessive bleeding as the midwives gained skills and confidence: the postpartum haemorrhage rate dropped from 21 per cent in the pilot study to 12 per cent in the first four months and during the last six months it was 7 per cent. It is also more common for women to have successful physiological births in birth centres and at home than in obstetric units (Brocklehurst *et al* 2011).

It seems to us from the research and the many reports we have that, whatever the problems of maternity care, enabling women and midwives to forge trusting relationships can only be helpful in trying to implement the changes we need to support all aspects of pregnancy, labour, birth and beyond. We need to find ways to increase women's knowledge and midwifery skills and move towards respecting and valuing physiological birth and women's abilities to know how best to do this. For physiological placental birth to become a real option for those women who want this, midwives need to be supported in their role and work. We would also need to relax the routine time limits on the birth of the placenta which currently are more appropriate for women having actively managed third stages, and start thinking more deeply about some of the wider issues that we have discussed in this book.

Until then, however you plan to labour and birth your baby and placenta (and remember that plans can change), we hope that this book has contributed to your knowledge, increased your confidence so that you are well enough informed to talk with your care provider, plan an environment that best supports you and make your own decisions.

References

ACOG (2016). Delayed umbilical cord clamping after birth. Committee Opinion Number 684.

Aflaifel N & Weeks AD (2012). Active management of the third stage of labour. British Medical Journal 2012:345: e4546.

Andersson O, Hellstrom-Westas L, Andersson D *et al* (2011). Effect of delayed versus early umbilical cord clamping on neonatal outcomes and iron status at 4 months. BMJ 2011 343: d7157.

Bais J, Eskes M, Pel M *et al* (2004). Postpartum haemorrhage in nulliparaous women: incidence and risk factors in low and high risk women. European Journal of Obstetrics & Gynecology and Reproductive Biology 115(2):166-72.

Baskett TF (2000). A flux of reds: evolution of active management of the third stage of labour. Journal of the Royal Society of Medicine 93(3): 489-493.

Beech BAL (2014). Am I Allowed? London: AIMS.

Begley CM (1990a). A comparison of 'active' and 'physiological' management of the third stage of labour. Midwifery 6(1): 3-17.

Begley CM (1990b). The effect of ergometrine on breastfeeding. Midwifery 6(2): 60-72.

Begley CM (2014). Intervention or interference? The need for expectant care throughout normal labour. Sexual and Reproductive Healthcare 5(4): 160-64.

Begley CM, Gyte GML, Devane D *et al* (2015). Active versus expect--ant management for women in the third stage of labour. Cochrane Database of Systematic Reviews 2015, Issue 3. Art. No.: CD007412.

Begley CM, Gyte GM, Murphy DJ *et al* (2010). Active versus expectant management for women in the third stage of labour. Cochrane Database of Systematic Reviews Issue 7.

Benyshek DC, Cheyney M, Brown J *et al* (2018). Placentophagy among women planning community births in the United States: Frequency, rationale, and associated neonatal outcomes. Birth doi: 10.1111/birt.12354. [Epub ahead of print].

Bhatt S, Alison BJ, Wallace EM *et al* (2013). Delaying cord clamping until ventilation onset improves cardiovascular function at birth in preterm lambs. The Journal of Physiology, 591(8), 2113-26.

Bloomfield TH, Gordon H (1990). Reaction to blood loss at delivery. Journal of Obstetrics and Gynaecology 10(Suppl 2): S13–S16.

Borovac-Pinheiro A, Pacagnella R, Cecatti J *et al* (2018). Postpartum hemorrhage: new insights for definition and diagnosis, American Journal of Obstetrics & Gynecology doi: 10.1016/j.ajog.2018.04.013.

Bose P, Regan F, Paterson-Brown S (2006). Improving the accuracy of estimated blood loss at obstetric haemorrhage using clinical reconstructions. British Journal of Obstetrics and Gynaecology 113(8): 919-24.

Botha MC (1968). The management of the umbilical cord in labour. South African Journal of Obstetrics and Gynaecology 16(2): 30-33.

Briley A, Seed PT, Tydeman G *et al* (2014). Reporting errors, incidence and risk factors for postpartum haemorrhage and progression to severe PPH: a prospective observational study. British Journal of Obstetrics and Gynaecology 121(7): 876-88.

Brocato B, Holliday N, Whitehurst RM *et al* (2016). Delayed cord clamping in preterm neonates: A review of benefits and risks. Obstetrical & Gynecological Survey, 71(1), 39-42.

Brocklehurst P, Hardy P, Hollowell J *et al.* (2011) Perinatal and maternal outcomes by planned place of birth for healthy women with low risk pregnancies: the Birthplace in England national prospective cohort study. British Medical Journal 343: d7400.

Buckley SJ (2005) Gentle Birth, Gentle Mothering. Brisbane: One Moon Press.

Buckley S (2009) Gentle birth, gentle mothering: a doctor's guide to natural childbirth and gentle early parenting choices. Celestial Arts. Several of Sarah's articles can be found at www.sarahbuckley.com

Buckley S (2011). Ask Away: Are there any psychophysiological benefits to women of physiological third stage management compared with active management of the third stage of labour? Essentially MIDIRS 2(3): 37-38.

Buckley SJ (2015). Hormonal physiology of childbearing: Evidence and implications for women, babies, and maternity care. Childbirth Connection Programs, National Partnership for Women & Families: Washington DC.

Burnley M, Roberts CL, Thatcher R (2006). Influence of blood donation on O2 uptake on kinetics, peak O2 uptake and time to exhaustion during severe-intensity cycle exercise in humans. Experimental Physiology 91: 499–509.

Chaparro CM, Neufeld LM, Tena Alavez G et al (2006). Effect of timing of umbilical cord clamping on iron status in Mexican infants: a randomised controlled trial. Lancet, 367(9527): 1997-2004.

Coyle CW, Hulse KE, Wisner KL et al (2015). Placentophagy: therapeutic miracle or myth? Archives of Women's Mental Health. 18(5): 673-80.

Cresswell JA, Ronsmans C, Calvert C et al (2013). Prevalence of placenta praevia by world region: a systematic review and meta-analysis. Tropical Medicine and International Health 18(6): 712-24.

Cronk M & Flint C (1989). Community Midwifery: A Practical Guide. Heinemann Medical Books. Chapter 4, 50-71.

Crowther S, Smythe E, Spence D (2015). Kairos time at the moment of birth. Midwifery 31: 451–457.

Darwin E (1801). Zoonomia: Or the laws of organic life. London.

Davies L (2007). Would you like a lotus birth with that ma'am? The increasing menu of choice and caesarean section. MIDIRS Midwifery Digest 17(4): 463-66.

Davies L (2011). Physiological third stage: how long is too long? Essentially MIDIRS 2(6): 38-42.

Davis D, Baddock S, Pairman S *et al* (2012). Risk of severe postpartum hemorrhage in low-risk childbearing women in New Zealand: exploring the effect of place of birth and comparing third stage management of labor. Birth. 39: 98–105.

Davis J (2010). Striking gorilla hormones, compelling circles and awesome plastic bag tricks: experiences of attending the Midatlantic conference on birth and primal health research. MIDIRS Midwifery Digest 20(2): 176-78.

Dixon L, Fletcher L, Tracy S *et al* (2009). Midwives care during the third stage of labour: An analysis of the New Zealand College of Midwives Midwifery Database 2004-2008. New Zealand College of Midwives Journal 41: 20-25.

Dixon L, Tracy SK, Guilliland K (2013). Outcomes of physiological and active third stage labour care amongst women in New Zealand. Midwifery. 29(1): 67-74.

Dunn PM (1989). Perinatal factors influencing adaptation to extrauterine life. Proceedings of the 12th World Congress Obstetrics and Gynecology, Rio de Janeiro. Parthenon Publishing 15: 119-123.

Dunn PM (1991). The third stage of labour and fetal adaptation at birth. Wyeth Guest Lecture. 1st International Congress of Perinatal Medicine. Tokyo, November 7 1991.

Dunn PM (2004). Clamping the umbilical cord. AIMS Journal 16(4): 8-9.

Dunn PM, Frazer ID, Raper AB (1966). Influence of early cord ligation on the transplacental passage of the foetal cells. Journal of Obstetrics & Gynaecology of the British Commonwealth 73: 757-60.

Edmunds J (1998). Hemorrhage: stay close and pay attention to your mothers. Midwifery Today 48: 14-16.

Edwards N & Wickham S (2011). Birthing Your Placenta: the third stage of labour. Third edition. AIMS.

Edwards N, Mander R, Murphy-Lawless J (2018). Untangling the maternity crisis. Abingdon: Routledge.

Fahy KM (2009). Third stage of labour care for women at low risk of postpartum haemorrhage. Journal of Midwifery and Women's Health 54(5): 380-86.

Fahy K, Hastie C, Bisits A *et al* (2010). Holistic physiological care compared to active management of the third stage of labour for women at low risk of postpartum haemorrhage: A cohort study. Women and Birth 23: 146-152.

Farr A, Chervenak FA, McCulloch LB *et al* (2016). Human placentophagy: a review. American Journal of Obstetrics and Gynecology 218(4): 401.e1-401.e11

Farrar D, Tuffnell D, Airey R *et al* (2010). Care during the third stage of labour: A postal survey of UK midwives and obstetricians. BMC Pregnancy and Childbirth 10:23.

Featherstone IE (1999). Physiological third stage of labour. British Journal of Midwifery 7(4): 216-221.

Fraser DM & Cooper MA (2003). Myles Textbook for Midwives. Edinburgh: Churchill Livingstone.

Fraser DM & Cooper MA (2009). Myles Textbook for Midwives. Edinburgh: Churchill Livingstone.

Foureur M (2008). Creating birth space to enable undisturbed birth. In: Fahy K, Foureur M, Hastie C (eds). Birth Territory and Midwifery Guardianship: Theory for Practice. Education and Research. Edinburgh: Books for Midwives 57-77.

Gallos ID, Williams HM, Price MJ *et al* (2018). Uterotonic agents for preventing postpartum haemorrhage: a network meta-analysis. Cochrane Database of Systematic Reviews 2018, Issue 4. Art. No.: CD011689.

Green JM, Coupland VA, Kitzinger JV (1998). Great expectations: a prospective study of women's expectations and experiences of childbirth. Oxford: Books for Midwives.

Grotegut CA, Paglia MJ, Johnson LNC *et al* (2011). Oxytocin exposure during labor among women with postpartum hemorrhage secondary to uterine atony. American Journal of Obstetrics and Gynecology 204(1): 56.e1-6.

Gülmezoglu AM, Forna F, Villar J *et al* (2007). Prostaglandins for preventing postpartum haemorrhage. Cochrane Database of Systematic Reviews 2007, Issue 3. Art. No.: CD000494.

Gülmezoglu AM, Lumbiganon P, Landoulsi S *et al* (2012). Active management of the third stage of labour with and without controlled cord traction: a randomised, controlled, non-inferiority trial. Lancet 379(9827): 1721-27. [Erratum appears in Lancet 379(9827):1704].

Gülmezoglu AM, Widmer M, Merialdi M *et al* (2009). Active management of the third stage of labour without controlled cord traction: a randomized non inferiority controlled trial. Reproductive Health 6(2).

Gurnsey J & Davies S (2010). A care pathway for the physiological third stage of labour. Essentially MIDIRS 1(4): 32-36.

Gyte G (1990). The Bristol third stage trial, Teachers' Broadsheet, New Generation 9(1): 29.

Gyte G (1991). The continuing debate on the third stage of labour. AIMS Journal 3(1): 4-6.

Gyte G (1992). The significance of blood loss at delivery. MIDIRS Midwifery Digest 2(1): 88-92.

Gyte G (1994). Evaluation of the meta-analysis on the effects on both mother and baby, of the various components of 'active management' of the third stage of labour. Midwifery 10: 183-99.

Hansen R, Gibson S, De paiva Alves E *et al* (2018). Adaptive response of neonatal sepsis-derived Group B Streptococcus to bilirubin. Scientific Reports. 8: 6470.

Harding JE, Elbourne DA, Prendiville PJ (1989). Views of mothers and midwives participating in the Bristol randomised trial of active management of the third stage of labour. Birth 16(1): 1-6.

Hastie C (2011). The birthing environment: a sustainable approach. In: Davies L, Daellenbach R, Kensington M (eds). Sustainability, Midwifery and Birth. Oxon: Routledge. 101-114.

Heller HT, Mullen KM, Gordon RW *et al* (2014). Outcomes of pregnancies with a low-lying placenta diagnosed on second-trimester sonography. Journal of Ultrasound Medicine 33(4): 691-96.

Hoffman M, Castagnola D, Naqvi F (2006). A randomized trial of active versus expectant management of the third stage of labor. American Journal of Obstetrics and Gynecology 195(6) Suppl 1: S107.

Hofmeyr G, Mshweshwe NT, Gülmezoglu A (2015). Controlled cord traction for the third stage of labour. Cochrane Database of Systematic Reviews 2015, Issue 1. Art. No.: CD008020.

Hofmeyr GJ, Neilson JP, Alfirec Z et al (2008). A Cochrane Pocketbook: Pregnancy and Childbirth. Chichester :Wiley.

Homer CSE, Leap N, Edwards N *et al* (2017). Midwifery continuity of carer in an area of high socio-economic disadvantage in London: a retrospective analysis of Albany Midwifery Practice outcomes using routine data 1997-2009. Midwifery 48: 1-10.

Hooper SB, Polglase GR, Te Pas AB (2015). A physiological approach to the timing of umbilical cord clamping at birth. Archives of Disease in Childhood - Fetal & Neonatal Edition 100(4), F355-360.

Hutchon DJ (2012). Immediate or early cord clamping vs delayed clamping. Journal of Obstetrics & Gynaecology, 32(8), 724-29.

Hutchon DJR (2016a). Strictly physiological neonatal transition at birth. Health Science Journal, 10(2), 1-3.

Hutchon DJR (2016b). Ventilation, chest compression and placental circulation at neonatal resuscitation – ILCOR recommendation 2015. Journal of Paedatric Neonatal Disorders 1(1): 1-6.

Hutchon DJR & Wepster R (2014). The estimated cost of early cord clamping at birth within Europe. International Journal of Childbirth, 4(4): 250-56.

Inch S (1983). Third stage management. ARM Newsletter 19: 7-8.

Inch S (1985). Management of the third stage of labour – another cascade of intervention? Midwifery 1(2): 114-122.

Inch S (1989). Birthrights. London: Greenprint.

Inch S (1990). Bristol third stage trial commentary. AIMS Journal 1(4): 8-10.

Jerbi M, Hidar S, Elmoueddeb S *et al* (2007). Oxytocin in the third stage of labor. International Journal of Gynecology and Obstetrics, 96(3): 198–99.

Jordan N (2017). Placenta Wit: mother stories, rituals and research. Demeter Press.

Jordan S, Emery S, Watkins A *et al* (2009). Associations of drugs routinely given in labour with breastfeeding at 48 hours: analysis of the Cardiff Births Survey. BJOG 116(12): 1622-32.

Kashanian M, Fekrat M, Masoomi Z *et al* (2010). Comparison of active and expectant management on the duration of the third stage of labour and the amount of blood loss during the third and fourth stage of labour. Midwifery 26(2): 241–45.

Khan GQ, John IS, Wani S *et al* (1997). Controlled cord traction versus minimal intervention techniques in delivery of the placenta: a randomised controlled trial. American Journal of Obstetrics and Gynecology 177(4): 770–74.

Kierse MJNC (1998). What does prevent postpartum haemorrhage? The Lancet, 351: 690-92.

Kirkham M (2018a). A Fundamental Contradiction: the business model does not fit midwifery values. Midwifery Matters 152: 13-15.

Kirkham M (2018b). Standardisation of care: a contradiction in terms. Midwifery Matters 157: 4-7.

Kitzinger S (2000). Rediscovering Birth. Pinter and Martin.

Knight M, Nair M, Tuffnell D *et al* for MBRRACE-UK (2017). Saving Lives, Improving Mothers' Care Lessons learned to inform maternity care from the UK and Ireland Confidential Enquiries into Maternal Deaths and Morbidity 2013–15. MBRRACE-UK.

Kroll-Desrosiers AR, Nephew BC, Babb JA *et al* (2017). Association of peripartum synthetic oxytocin administration and depressive and anxiety disorders within the first postpartum year. Depression & Anxiety 34(2): 137-46.

Lapido OA (1972). Management of third stage of labour with particular reference to reduction of feto-maternal transfusion. British Medical Journal 1(5802), 721–72.

Leung SW, Ng PS, Wong WY *et al* (2006). A randomised trial of carbetocin versus syntometrine in the management of the third stage of labour. BJOG: An International Journal of Obstetrics and Gynaecology 113(12): 1459-64.

Levy V (1990). The midwife's management of the third stage of labour. In: Alexander J, Levy V, Roch S (eds). Midwifery Practice: Intrapartum Care A Research Based Approach. London: Macmillan.

Levy V & Moore J (1985) The midwife's management of the third stage of labour. Nursing Times 81(5): 47-50.

Lim R (2015). Placenta: the forgotten chakra. 1st World Library.

Logue M (1990). Management of the third stage of labour: a midwife's view. Journal of Obstetrics and Gynaecology 10(S2):10-12.

Marchant S, Alexander J, Garcia J *et al* (1999). A survey of women's experiences of vaginal loss from 24 hours to three months after childbirth (the BLiPP study). Midwifery 15(2):72-81.

McCourt C (2013). Childbirth, Midwifery and Concepts of Time. London: Berghahn.

McDonald S (1999). Physiology and management of the third stage of labour. In: Bennett VR, Brown LK (eds). Myles Textbook for Midwives 13th edition. Edinburgh: Churchill Livingstone, 465-488.

McDonald S (2003). Physiology and management of the third stage of labour. In: Fraser DM, Cooper MA (eds). Myles Textbook for Midwives 14th edition. Edinburgh: Churchill Livingstone, 507-530.

McDonald SJ, Middleton P, Dowswell T *et al* (2013). Effect of timing of umbilical cord clamping of term infants on maternal and neonatal outcomes. Cochrane Database of Systematic Reviews 2013, Issue 7. Art. No.: CD004074. DOI: 10.1002/14651858.CD004074.pub3

McDonald S, Prendiville WJ, Elbourne DA (1999) Prophylactic syntometrine versus oxytocin for delivery of the placenta. The Cochrane Library, Issue 2, Oxford: Update Software.

Mercer JS (2001). Current best evidence: a review of the literature on umbilical cord clamping. Journal of Midwifery and Women's Health 46(6): 402–14.

Mercer J & Erickson-Owens D (2006) Delayed cord clamping increases infants' iron stores. Comment. Lancet 367(9527): 1956-58.

Mercer J & Erickson-Owens D (2010). Evidence for neonatal transition and the first hour of life. In: Walsh D, Downe S (eds). Essential midwifery practice: intrapartum care. Wiley, 81-104.

Mercer JS & Erickson-Owens DA (2014). Is it time to rethink cord management when resuscitation is needed? Journal of Midwifery & Women's Health, 59(6), 635-644.

Mercer JS, Erickson-Owens DA, Collins J *et al* (2017). Effects of delayed cord clamping on residual placental blood volume, hemoglobin and bilirubin levels in term infants: a randomized controlled trial. Journal of Perinatology 37: 260-64.

Mercer JS, Nelson CC, Skovgaard RL (2000). Umbilical cord clamping: beliefs and practices of American nurse-midwives. Journal of Midwifery and Women's Health 45(1): 58–66.

Mercer J, Skovgaard R, Erickson-Owens D (2008). Fetal to neonatal transition: first do no harm. In: Downe S (eds). Normal Childbirth: evidence and debate. Churchill Livingstone, 149–74.

Murphy-Lawless J (1998). Reading Birth and Death. A history of obstetric thinking. Cork University Press.

Muza S (2017). New Cochrane Review: Delayed cord clamping likely beneficial for healthy term newborns. https://tinyurl.com/ya5c3x9c

Ng PS, Chan ASM, Sin WK *et al* (2001). A multicentre randomized controlled trial of oral misoprostol and IM syntometrine in the management of the third stage of labour. Human Reproduction 16(1): 31-35.

NICE (2007). Intrapartum care: care of healthy women and their babies during childbirth. NICE clinical guideline 55.

NICE (2014). Intrapartum care for healthy women and babies. NICE Clinical Guideline 190.

NICE (2017a). Care in third stage of labour: NICE Pathway. https://pathways.nice.org.uk/pathways/intrapartum-care/care-in-third-stage-of-labour

NICE (2017b). Quality statement 6: Delayed cord clamping. www.nice.org.uk/guidance/qs105/chapter/quality-statement-6-delayed-cord-clamping

Nove A, Berrington A, Matthews Z (2012). Comparing the odds of postpartum haemorrhage in planned home birth against planned hospital birth: results of an observational study of over 500,000 maternities in the UK. BMC Pregnancy & Childbirth. 12: 130.

Novikova N, Hofmeyr G, Cluver C *et al* (2015). Tranexamic acid for preventing postpartum haemorrhage. Cochrane Database of Systematic Reviews 2015, Issue 6. Art. No.: CD007872.

NZCOM (2009). Third stage management practices of midwife lead maternity carers: an analysis of the New Zealand College of Midwives Midwifery Database Information 2004-2008. Christchurch: New Zealand College of Midwives.

Odent M (1998a). Physiological birth is normal birth. Midwifery Today Conference 'Keeping Birth Normal', London. Sept 10-14.

Odent M (1998b). Don't manage the third stage of labour! Practising Midwife 1(9): 31-33.

Odent M (1999). The Scientification of Love. London: Free Association books.

Odent M (2002). The first hour following birth: don't wake the mother. Midwifery Today 61: 9-11.

Page LA and McCandlish R (2006). The New Midwifery: Science and Sensitivity in Practice. London: Churchill Livingstone.

Porter M, MacIntyre S (1984). What is must be best: a research note on conservative or deferential responses to antenatal care provision. Social Science and Medicine 9(11): 1197-1200.

Positive Birth Movement (2018). https://tinyurl.com/yayrr7gr

Prendiville W & Elbourne D (1989). Care during the third stage of labour. In: Chalmers I, Enkin M, Kierse MJNC (eds). Effective Care in Pregnancy and Childbirth. Oxford University Press. 2: 1145-69.

Prendiville WJ, Elbourne DA, McDonald S (1999). Active versus expectant management of the third stage of labour. The Cochrane Library, Issue 2. Oxford: Update Software.

Prendiville WJ, Elbourne D, McDonald S (2000). Active versus expectant management in the third stage of labour. Cochrane Database of Systematic Reviews. Issue 3.

Prendiville WJ, Harding, JE, Elbourne DA *et al* (1988). The Bristol third stage trial: active versus physiological management of third stage labour. British Medical Journal 297: 1295-1300.

Prichard K, O'Boyle A, Hogden J (1995). Third stage of labour: outcomes of physiological third stage of labour care in the homebirth setting. New Zealand College of Midwives Journal April 1995: 8-10.

Raju TNK (2014). Delayed cord clamping: does gravity matter? The Lancet 384(9939):213-4.

Ramirez O, Benito V, Jimenez R *et al* (2001). Third stage of labour: active or expectant management? Journal of Perinatal Medicine 2001; Suppl 1(Pt 2), 364.

Rankin J (2017). Physiology in Childbearing: with Anatomy and Related Biosciences. Fourth edition. Oxford: Elsevier.

RANZCOG (2017). Provision of routine intrapartum care in the absence of pregnancy complications. https://tinyurl.com/yblp6p9z

Razvi K, Chua S, Arulkumaran S *et al* (1996). A comparison between visual estimation of laboratory determination of blood loss during the third stage of labour. Australian and New Zealand Journal of Obstetrics and Gynaecology 36(2): 152-54.

RCM (2008). Third Stage of Labour: Midwifery Practice Guideline. London: RCM, 2008.

RCOG (2015). Clamping of the Umbilical Cord and Placental Transfusion. Scientific Impact Paper No. 14. London: RCOG.

Robinson J (1999). Foreword. In Edwards N (1999). Delivering Your Placenta: The Third Stage. London: AIMS.

Rogers J & Wood J (1999). The Hinchingbrooke third stage trial: what are the implications for practice. Practising Midwife 2(2): 35-37.

Rogers J & Wood J (2003). The Hinchingbrooke third stage trial: In: Wickham S (Ed.) Midwifery Best Practice. Churchill Livingstone: London.

Rogers J, Wood J, McCandlish R *et al* (1998). Active versus expectant management of the third stage of labour: the Hinchingbrooke randomised controlled trial. The Lancet 351: 693-99.

Rosales-Ortiz S, Aguando RP, Hernandez RS *et al* (2014). Carbetocin versus oxytocin for prevention of postpartum haemorrhage: a randomised controlled trial. The Lancet 383: S51.

Sackett D (1996). Evidence based medicine: what it is and what it isn't. BMJ 312: 71-72.

Sandall J, Coxon K, Mackintosh N *et al* (2016). Relationships: the pathway to safe high-quality maternity care. Report from the Sheila Kitzinger symposium, Oxford. https://tinyurl.com/ybcw4d6t

Santalahti P *et al* (1998). On what grounds do women participate in prenatal screening? Prenatal Diagnosis 18(2): 153-65.

Schmid V (2005). About physiology in pregnancy and childbirth. Italy: Firenze.

Schorn MN (2010). Measurement of blood loss: review of the literature. Journal of Midwifery and Women's Health 55(1): 20-27.

Selfe K & Walsh DJ (2015). The third stage of labour: are low-risk women really offered an informed choice? MIDIRS Midwifery Digest 25(1): 66-72.

Sleep J (1989). Physiology and management of the third stage of labour. In: Bennett VR & Brown LK (eds). Myles Textbook for Midwives 11th edition. Edinburgh: Churchill Livingstone: 209-222.

Sleep J (1993). Physiology and management of the third stage of labour. In Bennet VR & Brown LK (eds). Myles Textbook for Midwives 12th edition. Edinburgh: Churchill Livingstone: 216-229.

SOGC (2015). Umbilical Cord Blood: Counselling, Collection, and Banking. SOGC Clinical Practice Guideline No. 328. Journal of Obstetrics & Gynaecology Canada. 37(9): 832–44.

Stevenson J (1989). The Bristol third stage trial. ARM Journal 4:11-12.

Stockdale H (1997). Over view of the management of the third stage of labour. Open Line 5(3): 9-10, 21-22.

Su LL, Rauff M, Chan YH *et al* (2009). Carbetocin versus syntometrine for the third stage of labour following vaginal delivery – a double-blind randomised controlled trial. BJOG: An International Journal of Obstetrics and Gynaecology 116(11): 1461-66.

Thilaganathan B, Cutner A, Latimer J (1993). Management of the third stage of labour in women at low risk of postpartum haemorrhage. European Journal of Obstetrics and Gynaecology and Reproductive Biology 48(1):19-22.

Thomas MR, Yoxall CW, Weeks AD *et al* (2014). Providing newborn resuscitation at the mother's bedside: assessing the safety, usability and acceptability of a mobile trolley. BMC Paediatrics 14: 135.

Tinson A, Ayrton C, Barker K *et al* (2016). Monitoring poverty and social exclusion 2016 (MPSE). New Policy Institute.

Urner F, Zimmerman R, Krafft A (2014). Manual Removal of the Placenta after Vaginal Delivery: An Unsolved Problem in Obstetrics. Journal of Pregnancy 2014: 274651.

Uvnäs Moberg K (2003). The Oxytocin Factor: Tapping the Hormone of Calm, Love and Healing. Da Capo Press.

Uvnäs Moberg K (2011). The Oxytocin Factor: Tapping the Hormone of Calm, Love and Healing. Pinter and Martin.

Vain NE, Satragno DS, Gorenstein AN *et al* (2014). Effect of gravity on volume of placental transfusion: a multicentre, randomised, non-inferiority trial. The Lancet 384(9939): 235-40.

van Dongen PWJ & de Groot ANJA (1995). History of ergot alkaloids from ergotism to ergometrine. European Journal of Obstetrics and Gynaecology and Reproductive Biology 60(2): 109-16.

van Teijlingen ER, Hundley V, Rennie AM *et al* (2003). Maternity Satisfaction Studies and their limitations: "What is must still be best". Birth 30(2): 75-82.

Vasegh FR, Bahiraie A, Mahmoudi M *et al* (2005). Comparison of active and physiologic management of third stage of labor. HAYAT: The Journal of Tehran Faculty of Nursing and Midwifery 10(23): 102.

Vincent-Priya J (1991). Birth without Doctors: Conversations with Traditional Midwives. Earthscan.

Vincent-Priya J (1992). Birth traditions and modern pregnancy care. Element Books.

Watson B (1990). A study of haemoglobin levels in women before and after childbirth. Midwives Chronicle 103(1228): 156-58.

Weeks A (2007). Editorial: Umbilical Cord Clamping After Birth. British Medical Journal 335: 312.

Wesson N (2006). Home Birth: A Practical Guide. Pinter and Martin.

WHO (1996). Care in normal birth: a practical guide, Report of a Technical Working Group. WHO/FRH /MSM/96.24, Geneva.

WHO (2012). WHO recommendations for the prevention and treatment of postpartum haemorrhage. Geneva: WHO. https://tinyurl.com/y7kbm5ms

WHO (2017). Optimal timing of cord clamping for the prevention of iron deficiency anaemia in infants. https://tinyurl.com/lwx7rap

Wickham S (1999). Further thoughts on the third stage. Practising Midwife 8(11): 37.

Wickham S (2001). Anti-D in Midwifery: Panacea or Paradox? Edinburgh: Books for Midwives.

Wickham S (2005). The birth of water embolism. Practising Midwife 8(11): 37.

Wickham S (2010). Research Unwrapped. Practising Midwife 3(2): 31-32.

Wickham S (2013). Top ten tips for facilitating physiological placental birth. Essentially MIDIRS 4(4): 27-31.

Wickham S (2015). Pondering Placentophagy: part 1. Practising Midwife 18(10): 60-62.

Wickham S (2018a). Inducing Labour: making informed decisions. Second Edition. Birthmoon Creations.

Wickham S (2018b). What's Right For Me? Making decisions in pregnancy and childbirth. Second Edition. Birthmoon Creations.

Wickham S (2018c). Group B Strep Explained. Second Edition. Birthmoon Creations, forthcoming.

Widmer M, Piaggio G, Nguyen TMH *et al* for the WHO CHAMPION Trial Group (2018). Heat-stable carbetocin vs oxytocin to prevent hemorrhage after vaginal birth. New England Journal of Medicine. www.nejm.org/doi/full/10.1056/NEJMoa1805489

Winter C, Macfarlane A, Deneux-Tharaux C *et al* (2007). Variations in policies for management of the third stage of labour and the immediate management of postpartum haemorrhage in Europe. British Journal of Obstetrics and Gynaecology 114(7): 845-54.

Wolford MC (1997). First do no harm. Midwifery Today 44: 15-17.

Yao AC & Lind J (1974). Placental transfusion. American Journal of Disease in Childhood. 127(1):128-41.

Zenack M (1998). Lotus Birth. Birthkit 18: 6.

Zinsser LA (2017). Lotus birth, a holistic approach on physiological cord clamping. Women and Birth 31(2):e73-e76.

Printed in Great Britain
by Amazon